SpringerBriefs in Statistics

For further volumes:
http://www.springer.com/series/8921

Hans-Michael Kaltenbach

A Concise Guide to Statistics

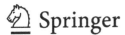 Springer

Dr. Hans-Michael Kaltenbach
ETH Zurich
Schwarzwaldallee 215
4002 Basel
Switzerland
e-mail: hans-michael.kaltenbach@bsse.ethz.ch

ISSN 2191-544X e-ISSN 2191-5458
ISBN 978-3-642-23501-6 e-ISBN 978-3-642-23502-3
DOI 10.1007/978-3-642-23502-3
Springer Heidelberg Dordrecht London New York

Library of Congress Control Number: 2011937427

Cover design: eStudio Calamar, Berlin/Figueres

Printed on acid-free paper

Springer is part of Springer Science+Business Media (www.springer.com)

To Elke

Preface

This book owes its existence to the lecture "Statistics for Systems Biology", which I taught in the fall semester 2010 at the Department for Biosystems Science and Engineering of the Swiss Federal Institute of Technology (ETH Zurich). To a large part, the audience consisted of students with backgrounds in biological sciences, which explains the large proportion of biological examples in this text.

Nevertheless, I hope that this text will be helpful for readers with very different backgrounds who need to quantify and analyze data to answer interesting questions. This book is not intended to be a manual, nor can it provide the answer to all questions and problems that one will encounter when analyzing data. Both the book title and the title of the book series indicate that space is limited and this book therefore concentrates more on the ideas and concepts rather than on presenting a vast array of different methods and applications. While all the standard material for an introductory course is covered, this text is very much inspired by Larry Wasserman's excellent book *All of Statistics* [1] and consequently discusses several topics usually not found in introductory texts, such as the bootstrap, robust estimators, and multiple testing, which are all found in modern statistics software. Due to the space constraints, this book does not cover methods from Bayesian statistics and does not provide any exercises. Frequent reference is made to the software R (freely available from http://www.r-project.org), but the text itself is largely independent from a particular software.

Should this book provide the reader with enough understanding of the fundamental concepts of statistics and thereby enable her or him to avoid some pitfalls in the analysis of data and interpretation of the results, such as by providing proper confidence intervals, not "accepting" a null hypothesis, or correcting for multiple testing where it is due, I shall be contented.

The book is organized in four chapters: Chapter 1 introduces the basics of probability theory, which allows to describe non-deterministic processes and is thus essential for statistics. Chapter 2 covers the inference of parameters and properties from given data, and introduces various types of estimators, their properties, and the computation of confidence intervals to quantify how good a given estimate is. Robust alternatives to important estimators are also provided.

Chapter 3 is devoted to hypothesis testing, with a main focus on the fundamental ideas and the interpretation of results. This chapter also contains sections on robust methods and correction for multiple testing, which become more and more important, especially in biology. Finally, Chap. 4 presents linear regression with one and several covariates and one-way analysis-of-variance. This chapter uses R more intensively to avoid tedious manual calculations, which the reader hopefully appreciates.

There surely is no shortage in statistics books. For further reading, I suggest to have a look at the two books by Wasserman: *All of Statistics* [1] and *All of Nonparametric Statistics* [2], which contain a much broader range of topics. The two books by Lehmann, *Theory of Point Estimation* [3] and *Testing Statistical Hypotheses* [4] contain almost everything one ever wanted to know about the material in Chaps. 2 and 3. For statistics using R, *Statistics—An Introduction using R* [5] by Crawley and *Introductory Statistics with R* [6] by Dalgaard are good choices, and *The R Book* [7] by Crawley offers a monumental reference. The *Tiny R Handbook* [8], published in the same series by Springer, might be a good companion to this book. For statistics related to bioinformatics, *Statistical Methods in Bioinformatics* [9] by Ewens and Grant provides lots of relevant information; the DNA sequence example is partly adapted from that book. Finally, for the german-speaking audience, I would recommend the two books by Pruscha *Statistisches Methodenbuch* [10], focusing on practical methods, and *Vorlesungen über mathematische Statistik* [11], its theory counterpart.

This script was typeset in LATEX, with all except the first two figures and all numerical data directly generated in R and included using Sweave [12].

I am indebted to many people that allowed this book to enter existence: I thank Jörg Stelling for his constant encouragement and support and for enabling me to work on this book. Elmar Hulliger, Ellis Whitehead, Markus Beat Dürr, Fabian Rudolf, and Robert Gnügge helped correcting various errors and provided many helpful suggestions. I thank my fiancée Elke Schlechter for her love and support. Financial support by the EU FP7 project UNICELLSYS is gratefully acknowledged. For all errors and flaws still lurking in the text, the figures, and the examples, I will nevertheless need to take full responsibility.

Basel, July 2011

Hans-Michael Kaltenbach

References

1. Wasserman, L.: All of Statistics. Springer, Heidelberg (2004)
2. Wasserman, L.: All of Nonparametric Statistics. Springer, Heidelberg (2006)
3. Lehmann, E.L., Casella, G.: Theory of Point Estimation, 2nd edn. Springer, Heidelberg (1998)
4. Lehmann, E.L., Romana, J.P.: Testing Statistical Hypotheses, 3rd edn. Springer, Heidelberg (2005)
5. Crawley, M.J.: Statistics—An Introduction using R. Wiley, New York (2005)

6. Dalgaard, R.: Introductory Statistics with R, 2nd edn. Springer, Heidelberg (2008)
7. Crawley, M.J.: The R Book. Wiley, New York (2007)
8. Allerhand, M.: A Tiny Handbook of R. Springer, Heidelberg (2011)
9. Ewens, W.J., Grant, G.R.: Statistical Methods in Bioinformatics. Springer, Heidelberg (2001)
10. Pruscha, H.: Statistisches Methodenbuch. Springer, Heidelberg (2006)
11. Pruscha, H.: Vorlesungen über Mathematische Statistik. Springer, Heidelberg (2000)
12. Leisch, F.: Sweave: Dynamic generation of statistical reports. In: Härdle, W., Rönz, B. (eds.) Compstat 2002—Proceedings in Computational Statistics, pp 575–580 (2002)

Contents

Chapter 1
Basics of Probability Theory

Abstract Statistics deals with the collection and interpretation of data. This chapter
lays a foundation that allows to rigorously describe non-deterministic processes and
to reason about non-deterministic quantities. The mathematical framework is given
by probability theory, whose objects of interest are random quantities, their description and properties.

Keywords Probability · Distribution · Moment · Quantile

> The laws of probability. So true in general. So fallacious in
> particular
>
> Edward Gibbon

1.1 Probability and Events

In statistics, we are concerned with the collection, analysis, and interpretation of
data, typically given as a random sample from a large set. We therefore need to
lay a foundation in probability theory that allows us to formally represent non-
deterministic processes and study their properties.

A first example. Let us consider the following situation: a dice is rolled leading
to any of the numbers $\{1, \ldots, 6\}$ as a possible *outcome*. With two dice, the possible
outcomes are described by the set

$$\Omega = \{(i, j)|1 \leq i, j \leq 6\},$$

of size $|\Omega| = 36$. The set of outcomes that lead to a sum of at least 10 is then

$$A = \{(4, 6), (6, 4), (5, 5), (5, 6), (6, 5), (6, 6)\} \subset \Omega,$$

a set of size 6. A first definition of the *probability* that we will roll a sum of at least
10 is given by counting the number of outcomes that lead to a sum larger or equal

H.-M. Kaltenbach, *A Concise Guide to Statistics*, SpringerBriefs in Statistics,
DOI: 10.1007/978-3-642-23502-3_1, © Hans-Michael Kaltenbach 2012

10 and divide it by the number of all possible outcomes:

$$\mathbb{P}(A) = \frac{|A|}{|\Omega|} = \frac{6}{36},$$

with the intuitive interpretation that 6 out of 36 possible outcomes are of the desired type. This definition implicitly assumes that each of the 36 possible outcomes has the same chance of occurring.

Any collection of possible outcomes $X \subseteq \Omega$ is called an *event*; the previous definition assigns a probability of $\mathbb{P}(X) = |X|/|\Omega|$ to such an event. Events are sets and we can apply the usual operations on them: Let A be as above the event of having a sum of at least 10. Let us further denote by B the event that both dice show an even number; thus, $B = \{(2, 2), (2, 4), (2, 6), (4, 2), (4, 4), (4, 6), (6, 2), (6, 4), (6, 6)\}$ and $|B| = 9$. The event C of rolling a sum of at least 10 *and* both dice even is then described by the *intersection* of the two events:

$$C = A \cap B = \{(4, 6), (6, 4), (6, 6)\},$$

and has probability

$$\mathbb{P}(C) = \mathbb{P}(A \cap B) = \frac{3}{36}.$$

Similarly, we can ask for the event of rolling a total of at least ten *or* both dice even. This event corresponds to the *union* of A and B, since any of the elements of A or B will do:

$$D := A \cup B = \{(5, 5), (5, 6), (6, 5), (2, 2), (2, 4), (2, 6),$$
$$(4, 2), (4, 4), (4, 6), (6, 2), (6, 4), (6, 6)\}.$$

The *complement* of an event corresponds to all possible outcomes that are not covered by the event itself. For example, the event of not rolling an even number simultaneously on both dice is given by the complement of B, which is

$$B^{\mathscr{C}} = \Omega \backslash B = \{(i, j) \in \Omega | (i, j) \notin B\},$$

with probability

$$\mathbb{P}\left(B^{\mathscr{C}}\right) = 1 - \mathbb{P}(B) = 1 - \frac{9}{36} = \frac{27}{36}.$$

The general case. Let Ω be the set of all possible outcomes of a particular experiment and denote by $A, B \subseteq \Omega$ any pair of events. Then, any function $\mathbb{P}$ with the properties

$$\mathbb{P}(\Omega) = 1, \tag{1.1}$$

$$\mathbb{P}(A) \geq 0, \tag{1.2}$$

$$\mathbb{P}(A \cup B) = \mathbb{P}(A) + \mathbb{P}(B) \text{ if } A \cap B = \emptyset \tag{1.3}$$

defines a *probability measure* or simply a *probability* that allows to compute the probability of events. The first requirement (1.1) ensures that Ω is really the set of all possible outcomes, so any experiment will lead to an element of Ω; the probability that *something* happens should thus be one. The second requirement (1.2) is that probabilities are never negative (but the probability of events might be zero). Finally, the third requirement (1.3) gives us the algebraic rule how the probability of combined events is computed; importantly, this rule only applies for disjoint sets. Using the algebra of sets as above, we can immediately derive some additional facts:

$$\mathbb{P}\left(A^{\mathscr{C}}\right) = \mathbb{P}(\Omega \backslash A) = 1 - \mathbb{P}(A),$$
$$\mathbb{P}(\emptyset) = 1 - \mathbb{P}(\Omega) = 0,$$
$$A \subseteq B \Rightarrow \mathbb{P}(A) \leq \mathbb{P}(B).$$

Importantly, there are multiple ways to define a valid probability measure for any given set Ω, so these three requirements do not specify a unique such measure. For assigning a probability to discrete events like the ones discussed so far, it is sufficient to specify the probability $\mathbb{P}(\{\omega\})$ for each possible outcome $\omega \in \Omega$ of the experiment. For example, a die is described by its outcomes $\Omega = \{1, 2, 3, 4, 5, 6\}$. One possible probability measure is $\mathbb{P}(\{\omega\}) = 1/6$ for each of the six possible outcomes ω; it describes a fair die. Another probability is $\mathbb{P}(\{1\}) = \mathbb{P}(\{3\}) = P(\{5\}) = 1/18$, $\mathbb{P}(\{2\}) = \mathbb{P}(\{4\}) = \mathbb{P}(\{6\}) = 2/18$, in which case the probability to roll an even number is twice the probability to roll an odd one. Both probability measures are valid, and the particular choice depends on the various assumptions that are made when modeling the die and its behavior.

Typically, probability measures are either derived from such assumptions or they are inferred from observed data. Such inference will be covered in Chap. 2. For more complex examples, it might not be straightforward to construct a probability measure that correctly captures all assumptions.

If the possible outcomes Ω become a continuous set, describing a length, for example, it is no longer possible to simply assign a probability to each element of this set to define a probability measure. This case requires more sophisticated mathematical machinery and is not covered here. However, the following results are essentially the same for discrete and continuous cases.

Union of events. We still need to delve a little deeper into the computation of event probabilities. Note that the probability for a union of events is only the sum of the two individual probabilities provided the two events do not overlap and there is no

Fig. 1.1 Venn diagram of
the sets A and B. To compute
the size of the union, the
"doubly-counted"
intersection $A \cap B$ has to be
subtracted once

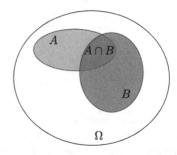

outcome that belongs to both events. In the above example of events A (sum larger
equal 10) and B (both dice even), this is clearly not the case. Consequently, the size
of their union D is smaller than the sum of the individual sizes of A and B.

For computing the probability of D from A and B, we can use an *inclusion-
exclusion* argument: The size of D is the size of A plus the size of B, minus the size
of the intersection $A \cap B$. This becomes clear if we draw a Venn-diagram of the sets
as in Fig. 1.1. The elements in the intersection are counted twice and we therefore
have to correct by subtracting it once. Indeed,

$$|D| = |A| + |B| - |A \cap B|,$$

and thus

$$\mathbb{P}(D) = \frac{|A|}{|\Omega|} + \frac{|B|}{|\Omega|} - \frac{|A \cap B|}{|\Omega|} = \mathbb{P}(A) + \mathbb{P}(B) - \mathbb{P}(A \cap B).$$

Note that if $A \cap B = \emptyset$, we recover the case (1.3) given in the original definition.

The inclusion–exclusion calculation is also possible for more than two sets, but
does get a little more involved: already for three sets, we now count some subsets
twice and three times.

Independence. One of the most important concepts in probability and statistics is
independence. Two events X and Y are independent if the knowledge that Y already
occurred does not influence the probability that X will occur. In other words, knowing
that Y happened gives us no information on whether X also happened or not, and vice-
versa.

As an example, let us again look at rolling two dice: with some justification, we
may assume that the roll of the first die does not influence the roll of the second. In
particular, it does not matter whether we roll both dice at once or roll the first and
then roll the second. In this example, the independence of the two dice is a modeling
assumption and other modeling assumptions are possible.

Formally, two events X and Y are independent if

$$\mathbb{P}(X \cap Y) = \mathbb{P}(X)\mathbb{P}(Y),$$

which means that the probability that both X and Y occur is the probability that X
occurs times the probability that Y occurs.

In the dice example, the event $E = \{(i, j)|i \geq 5\}$ of rolling a 5 or 6 on the first die, and $F = \{(i, j)|j \geq 5\}$ of rolling a 5 or 6 on the second die, are independent. Indeed, $\mathbb{P}(E \cap F) = \mathbb{P}(\{(i, j)|i \geq 5, j \geq 5\}) = \mathbb{P}(\{(5, 5), (5, 6), (6, 5), (6, 6)\}) = \frac{4}{36}$ and $\mathbb{P}(E) = \mathbb{P}(F) = \frac{2}{6}$.

If two events are not independent, the probability of X happening provided we already know that Y happened is captured by the *conditional probability* of X given Y, which we denote by $\mathbb{P}(X|Y)$. This probability is given by

$$\mathbb{P}(X|Y) = \frac{\mathbb{P}(X \cap Y)}{\mathbb{P}(Y)},$$

and might be easier to remember in its equivalent form $\mathbb{P}(X|Y)\mathbb{P}(Y) = \mathbb{P}(X \cap Y)$, which reads "the probability of X and Y happening simultaneously is the probability that Y happens times the probability that X happens if Y happened". For example, what is the probability to roll at least a total of 10, if we already know that both dice are even? There are $|B| = 9$ possible outcomes that lead to both dice even. From these, $|A \cap B| = 3$ have a sum of 10 or greater, leading to the probability

$$\mathbb{P}(A|B) = \frac{\mathbb{P}(A \cap B)}{\mathbb{P}(B)} = \frac{\frac{3}{36}}{\frac{9}{36}} = \frac{3}{9}.$$

If two events X and Y are independent, we have

$$\mathbb{P}(X|Y) = \mathbb{P}(X),$$

as we would expect. This also agrees with the above interpretation: The probability of X happening is the same, irrespective of knowing whether Y happened or not.

The *law of total probability* states that

$$\mathbb{P}(X) = \mathbb{P}(X \cap Y_1) + \cdots + \mathbb{P}(X \cap Y_n),$$

where the Y_i form a partition of Ω, i.e., cover all possible outcomes without covering one outcome twice. We can read this as "the probability that X happens is the probability that X and Y_1 happen simultaneously or X and Y_2 happen simultaneously etc.". The example in Fig. 1.2 gives an intuitive representation of the theorem.

Together, conditional probabilities and the law of total probability are powerful tools for computing the probability of particular events.

Example 1 Let us consider an urn containing 2 white and 3 black balls, from which two balls are drawn, and are not put back in (this is known as drawing without replacement). Let us denote by C the event that we draw two identical colors, no matter which one, and by W and B the event of the first ball being white, respectively black. Provided we know the first ball is white, we can conclude that there are 1 white and 3 black balls left in the urn. The probability to draw another white ball thus became

$$\mathbb{P}(C|W) = 1/4.$$

Fig. 1.2 Law of total
probability: $\mathbb{P}(X) =$
$\mathbb{P}(X \cap Y_1) + \cdots + \mathbb{P}(X \cap Y_n)$
if the Y_i partition Ω

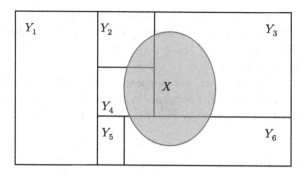

Similarly, if we know the first ball is black, we can conclude 2 white and 2 black balls being left and thus

$$\mathbb{P}(C|B) = 2/4.$$

By the law of total probability, $\mathbb{P}(C)$ is the probability to draw another white ball if we have a white, times the probability to draw a white in the first place plus the same for black:

$$\mathbb{P}(C) = \mathbb{P}(C \cap W) + \mathbb{P}(C \cap B) = \mathbb{P}(C|W)\mathbb{P}(W) + \mathbb{P}(C|B)\mathbb{P}(B).$$

With $\mathbb{P}(W) = 2/5$ and $\mathbb{P}(B) = 3/5$ this amounts to $\mathbb{P}(C) = 2/5$.

Bayes' rule. Bayes' rule is an important tool for manipulating conditional probabilities. It allows us to "invert" conditional probabilities by

$$\mathbb{P}(Y|X) = \mathbb{P}(X|Y)\frac{\mathbb{P}(Y)}{\mathbb{P}(X)} , \qquad (1.4)$$

which becomes evident if we simply multiply by $\mathbb{P}(X)$ to arrive at $\mathbb{P}(Y \cap X) = \mathbb{P}(X \cap Y)$. The two probabilities for X and Y are called the *prior* probabilities, as they describe the chance that either event happens without taking into account any information about the other event. The left-hand side of (1.4) is called the *posterior*. While algebraically simple, this rule is very helpful in computing conditional probabilities in a variety of situations.

Example 2 Let us consider the following situation: a patient is going to see a doctor for an annual checkup and in the battery of tests that are performed, the test for a particular disease D comes back positive. The doctor is concerned, as he read in the brochure that this particular test has a probability of 0.9 to correctly detect the disease if the patient actually has it, and also a probability of 0.9 to correctly detect if the patient does not have it. Should the patient be concerned, too?

Let us denote by $+$ and $-$ the events of positive, respectively negative, outcome of the test. From the brochure information, we know that

$$\mathbb{P}(+|D) = 0.9,$$
$$\mathbb{P}(-|D^{\mathscr{C}}) = 0.9.$$

But what we are really interested in is the probability $\mathbb{P}(D|+)$ that the patient actually has the disease, provided the test says so. We compute this probability via Bayes' rule as

$$\mathbb{P}(D|+) = \mathbb{P}(+|D)\frac{\mathbb{P}(D)}{\mathbb{P}(+)}.$$

We would therefore need to know the probability $\mathbb{P}(D)$ that a patient has the disease in the first place (regardless of any test results) and the probability $\mathbb{P}(+)$ that the test will be positive (regardless of whether the patient is sick). The latter is easily computed using the law of total probability

$$\mathbb{P}(+) = \mathbb{P}(+|D)\mathbb{P}(D) + \mathbb{P}(+|D^{\mathscr{C}})\mathbb{P}(D^{\mathscr{C}}),$$

and

$$\mathbb{P}(+|D^{\mathscr{C}}) = 1 - \mathbb{P}(-|D^{\mathscr{C}}).$$

The only thing we need to figure out is $\mathbb{P}(D)$, the probability to be sick in the first place. We might imagine this as the probability that, randomly picking someone from the street, this person is actually sick. It is important to understand that this probability has to be provided from the outside, as it cannot be derived from the information available in the problem specification. In our case, such data might be available from public health institutions. Let us assume that 1 in 100 people are sick, so $\mathbb{P}(D) = 0.01$ and consequently

$$\mathbb{P}(+) = 0.9 \times 0.01 + (1 - 0.9) \times (1 - 0.01) = 0.108,$$

that is, for about one out of ten people, the test will be positive, irrespective of their actual health. This is simply because few people have the disease, but in one out of ten, the test will be incorrect. We assembled all information needed to actually compute the relevant probability:

$$\mathbb{P}(D|+) = 0.9 \times \frac{0.01}{0.108} \approx 0.08.$$

Maybe surprisingly, the probability to have the disease if the test is positive is less that 10% and getting a second opinion is clearly indicated! This is one reason to perform a second *independent* test in such a case.

The key point of this example is to not get confused by the two conditional probabilities $\mathbb{P}(X|Y)$ and $\mathbb{P}(Y|X)$ and mistakenly assume them to be equal or at least of comparable size. As shown, the two can be very different, depending on the prior probabilities for X and Y.

Implications of Bayes' rule. Bayes' rule has some more implications along these lines, which we will briefly describe in a very informal manner: As we will see in the chapter on statistical hypothesis testing, classical techniques only allow us to compute the probability of seeing certain data D (e.g., a measurement), provided a given hypothesis H is true; very informally, $\mathbb{P}(D|H)$. Of course, we actually want to know the probability $\mathbb{P}(H|D)$ of the hypothesis being true, given the data. However, Bayes' rule shows that this probability can only be computed if we have information about the hypothesis being true irrespective of any data. Again, this information about prior probabilities has to come from "outside" and cannot be inferred from the hypothesis or the data. Typically, this information is provided by either additional assumptions or by looking into other data. The branch of Bayesian Statistics deals with the incorporation of such prior data and provides many alternative ways of inference and hypothesis testing. However, many of these methods are more elaborate and special care needs to be taken to correctly apply them, which is one reason why we do not cover them in this text.

1.2 Random Variables

While events and algebraic set operations form the basis for describing random experiments, we gain much more flexibility and widen the applications of probability by introducing *random variables*. Technically, these are functions mapping an outcome $\omega \in \Omega$ to a number. For example, we can describe the two dice example simply by defining the number of eyes rolled with die i as the random variable X_i. The event of having at least a 5 on the first die is then described intuitively by the statement $X_1 \geq 5$. Similarly, we can formulate the event that the sum is larger than 10 by $X_1 + X_2 \geq 10$, instead of listing all corresponding outcomes.

Once probabilities are assigned to events, they transfer to random variables simply by finding the corresponding event described by a statement on the random variables. Formally, $\mathbb{P}(X \in \mathscr{X}) = \mathbb{P}(\{\omega | X(\omega) \in \mathscr{X}\})$.

For the two dice example, let us compute the probability of rolling at least a 5 with the first die using the random variable X_1:

$$\begin{aligned}
\mathbb{P}(X_1 \geq 5) &= \mathbb{P}(X_1 \in \{5, 6\}) = \mathbb{P}(\{\omega \in \Omega | X_1(\omega) \in \{5, 6\}\}) \\
&= \mathbb{P}(\{(i, j) | i \geq 5, 1 \leq j \leq 6\}) \\
&= \mathbb{P}(\{(i, j) | i = 5\}) + \mathbb{P}(\{(i, j) | i = 6\}) = \frac{12}{36}.
\end{aligned}$$

The *joint probability* of two random variables X and Y simultaneously taking values in their respective sets is given by the intersection of the corresponding events:

$$\mathbb{P}(X \in \mathscr{X}, Y \in \mathscr{Y}) = \mathbb{P}(\{\omega | X(\omega) \in \mathscr{X}\} \cap \{\omega | Y(\omega) \in \mathscr{Y}\}).$$

The advantage of working with random variables instead of events comes from the fact that random variables have a *probability distribution* that describes the probability that the random variable takes a value smaller or equal to a certain number. The *cumulative distribution function (cdf)* $F_X()$ of a random variable X is defined as $F_X(x) = \mathbb{P}(X \leq x)$. It always starts with a value of 0 at $x = -\infty$ and monotonically increases to 1 for larger values of x. Often, very different problems lead to the same distribution for the involved random variables, which is why some distributions get their own name and their properties can be found in tables.

Similar to events, random variables also come in two distinct flavors: they either take values in a discrete (but maybe infinite) set of values, as in the dice example, or they take values from a continuous set, like the set of real numbers $\mathbb{R}$

Discrete Random Variables. A discrete random variable A has a *probability mass function (pmf)* in addition to its cumulative distribution function. The pmf is given by $p_A(a) = \mathbb{P}(A = a)$ and we can easily compute the cdf from it by summation: $F_A(k) = \sum_{a=-\infty}^{k} p_A(a)$.

Example 3 Let us consider the following experiment: a coin is flipped n times. The probability of any flip to show head is given by our first distribution with its own name: the *Bernoulli distribution*, which assigns a probability of p to head and $1 - p$ to tail. If X_i is the outcome of the ith flip, with $X_i = 0$ for tail and $X_i = 1$ for head, this distribution is completely described by p, as $\mathbb{P}(X_i = 0) = 1 - p$, $\mathbb{P}(X_i = 1) = p$ and $\mathbb{P}(X_i = k) = 0$ for any value k that is neither 0 nor 1. Thus, knowing that X_i is Bernoulli distributed with parameter p completely specifies all we need to know. In short, this statement is written as $X \sim \text{Bernoulli}(p)$, where "$\sim$" is read as "distributed as".

What is the probability that we have to wait until the wth flip to see head for the first time? This is the question for the distribution of a *waiting time* W. Let us see: to see the first head at flip w, all preceding $w - 1$ flips are necessarily tails. Assuming the flips to be independent, this probability is

$$\mathbb{P}(X_1 = 0, \ldots, X_{w-1} = 0) = \mathbb{P}(X_1 = 0) \cdots \mathbb{P}(X_{w-1} = 0) = (1 - p)^{w-1}.$$

The probability to actually see head in the wth flip is $\mathbb{P}(X_w = 1) = p$. Thus, $\mathbb{P}(W = w) = (1 - p)^{w-1} p$, the pmf of a *geometric distribution*, denoted $W \sim \text{Geom}(p)$. The particular value w is called a *realization* of the random variable W. This is an example of a discrete random variable that has infinitely many possible values with positive probability. The probability mass function of a geometric distribution is given in Fig. 1.3 (left).

What is the probability to see exactly h heads if we flip n times? This question is a little more tricky: the probability to see h heads in n flips is p^h. The probability that the remaining $n - h$ flips are all tails is $(1-p)^{n-h}$. But there are a multitude of ways to arrange the h heads and $n - h$ tails. To be exact, there are $\binom{n}{h} := \frac{n!}{(n-h)!h!}$ (a binomial coefficient, read "n choose h") many ways to do so: $n! := 1 \times 2 \times 3 \times \cdots \times n$ is the number of ways to arrange n flips in different order. The h heads can be drawn in $h!$

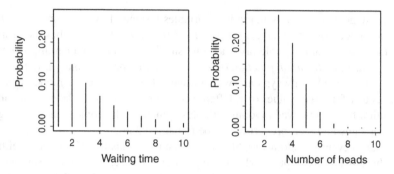

Fig. 1.3 Geometric distribution for $p = 0.3$ (*left*) and binomial distribution with $n = 10$ and $p = 0.3$ (*right*)

different orders, which we do not distinguish and treat as equivalent. Similarly, there are $(n - h)!$ ways to arrange the tails are equivalent, leading to the stated coefficient. More generally, the binomial coefficient gives the number of different ways to draw h objects out of n, if we do not care for the order in which they are drawn. For $n = 3$, there are $\binom{3}{2} = 3$ ways to draw exactly two of them: from the set $\{a, b, c\}$, the 3 ways are $\{a, b\}$, $\{b, c\}$, $\{a, c\}$. The first set contains two possible ways to draw: first the a, then the b, or vice-versa, and similarly for the other two sets.

For our problem, let H be the number of heads in n flips. This is a random variable taking values between 0 and n. It has a *binomial distribution* with two parameters n and p and probabilities given by the mass function

$$\mathbb{P}(H = h) = \binom{n}{h} (1 - p)^{n-h} p^{h};$$

denoted by $H \sim \text{Binom}(n, p)$. A plot of a binomial probability mass function is given in Fig. 1.3 (right).

Let us combine these two calculations of the waiting time and the number of heads by solving the following problem: again, a coin is flipped n times, the probability to see head is p. Let again H be the number of heads in these n flips and let W be the waiting time for the first head to appear. For completeness, we set $W = n + 1$, if no head appears at all.

What is the probability to simultaneously see h heads with the first head appearing at the wth flip? This questions asks for the joint probability distribution given by $\mathbb{P}(H = h, W = w)$.

The two random variables H, W are not independent: if they were, we would have $\mathbb{P}(H = h | W = w) = \mathbb{P}(H = h)$. But if no head has appeared at all (so $W = n + 1$), then the probability to see any more than zero heads, given this information, is zero: $\mathbb{P}(H = 1 | W = n + 1) = 0$, but $\mathbb{P}(H = 1) > 0$. For working out the correct answer, we therefore need to take this dependency into account. It is always a good idea to check some boundary cases first: as we saw,

Table 1.1 Joint probability distribution of (H, W)

	$w=1$	$w=2$	$w=3$	$w=4$
$h=0$	0.000	0.000	0.000	0.125
$h=1$	0.125	0.125	0.125	0.000
$h=2$	0.250	0.125	0.000	0.000
$h=3$	0.125	0.000	0.000	0.000

$$\mathbb{P}(H = 0, W = n+1) = \mathbb{P}(H = 0|W = n+1)\mathbb{P}(W = n+1) = 1 \times (1-p)^n,$$

the probability to see n tails. Further, $\mathbb{P}(H = 0, W = w) = 0$ for any $w \leq n$, as we cannot have seen the first head somewhere in the sequence if we saw none at all.

What about the non-boundary cases? For $(H = h, W = w)$, we can use the following argument: to see h heads in total, given the first one in the wth flip, we know that the first $w - 1$ flips are all tails and we need to place $h - 1$ heads in the remaining $n - w$ positions (the first is already placed in position w):

$$\mathbb{P}(H = h|W = w) = \binom{n-w}{h-1} (1-p)^{(n-w)-(h-1)} p^{h-1},$$

the binomial probability of having $h - 1$ heads in $n - w$ trials. The probability of first head at $w \leq n$ is the geometric distribution $\mathbb{P}(W = w) = (1-p)^{w-1}p$. Combining:

$$\mathbb{P}(H = h, W = w) = \binom{n-w}{h-1} (1-p)^{n-h} p^h.$$

The conditional distribution of waiting w flips, given we have h heads in total, is easily calculated as

$$\mathbb{P}(W = w|H = h) = \frac{\binom{n-w}{h-1}}{\binom{n}{h}},$$

the number of ways to place $h - 1$ heads in $n - w$ positions over the number of ways to place h heads in n positions. Interestingly, this probability is independent of the probability p to see head. For $n = 3$ and $p = 0.5$, the full joint probability $\mathbb{P}(H = h, W = w)$ is given in Table 1.1.

We might also be interested in computing the waiting time distribution without referring to the number of heads. This *marginal distribution* can be derived by applying the law of total probability. For example,

$$\mathbb{P}(W = 2) = \sum_{h=0}^{3} \mathbb{P}(H = h, W = 2) = (1-p)p = \frac{1}{4}$$

is the marginal probability that we see the first head in the second flip.

Example **4** To contribute another example, let us consider the following problem, encountered in molecular biology: DNA molecules carrying the inheritance information of an organism can be modeled as a sequence of nucleotides. There are four different such nucleotides: arginine (abbreviated A), cytosine (C), guanine (G), and tyrosine (T). A common problem is to determine how closely related two DNA sequences are. To make things easier, let us assume both sequences have the same length n, that the nucleotides in any two positions in the sequence are independent, and that each nucleotide has a probability of 1/4 to occur in any position. Similarity of the sequences can then be established by counting in how many positions the two sequences have the same nucleotide. Each such case is called a *match*, the converse a *mismatch*, so the following two sequences have seven matches and three mismatches (underlined):

$$A \ C \ \underline{C} \ G \ T \ T \ \underline{G} \ \underline{G} \ \underline{T} \ A$$
$$A \ C \ \underline{G} \ G \ T \ T \ \underline{C} \ G \ \underline{A} \ A$$

If the two sequences have nothing in common, we would expect to see a match in about 1/4 of the cases, and the number of matches would follow a Binom($n, p = 1/4$) distribution. Conversely, evolutionarily related DNA sequences would show a much higher proportion of matches.

In subsequent chapters, we will *estimate* the nucleotide frequencies p from data and *test the hypothesis* that sequences are related by comparing the observed and expected number of matches

Continuous Random Variables. We also need random variables that take values in a continuous set to describe, e.g., measured lengths or optical densities. Similar to events, we cannot cover these in all mathematical rigor. A nontrivial mathematical argument shows that for such a continuous random variables X, a probability mass function cannot be defined properly, because $\mathbb{P}(X = x) = 0$ for all x. Instead, most of these variables have a *probability density function (pdf)* $f_X(x)$ with the properties

$$f_X(x) \geq 0 \, ,$$

$$\int\limits_{-\infty}^{\infty} f_X(y)\mathrm{d}y = 1.$$

The density is a function such that the probability of X to take a value in any interval $[x_l, x_u]$ is given by the area under the density function on this interval, that is, $\mathbb{P}(x_l \leq X \leq x_u) = \int_{x_l}^{x_u} f_X(y)\mathrm{d}y$. This probability can also be written in terms of the cumulative distribution function

$$F_X(x) = \mathbb{P}(X \leq x) = \int\limits_{-\infty}^{x} f_X(y)\mathrm{d}y$$

Fig. 1.4 Density of Exp(λ) distribution for $\lambda = 2$. The gray shaded area gives the probability of W falling in the range [0.5, 2]

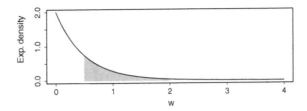

as the difference $F_X(x_u) - F_X(x_l)$. Important continuous distributions include the exponential (see Ex. 5 below) and the normal distributions (covered in Sect. 1.3). In Sect. 1.4, we will discuss several more distributions that frequently arise in statistics, like the t-, the χ^2- and the F-distributions, and also demonstrate various relations between them.

Example 5 As a first example for a continuous random variable, let us consider the *exponential distribution*. This distribution often describes the waiting time W for an event such as a radioactive decay and has density function

$$f_W(w; \lambda) = \lambda \exp(-\lambda w),$$

where the rate $\lambda > 0$ is the distribution's only parameter and $1/\lambda$ describes the average waiting time for the next event. The cumulative distribution function is easily calculated as

$$F_W(w; \lambda) = 1 - \exp(-\lambda w).$$

Figure 1.4 shows the density function for $\lambda = 2$, the area of the gray region gives the probability that a random variable $W \sim \text{Exp}(2)$ takes a value between 0.5 and 2, which we calulate to be

$$\mathbb{P}(0.5 \leq W \leq 2) = \int_{0.5}^{2} 2 \times \exp(-2 \times w)dw = 0.3496.$$

Example 6 Another example for a continuous distribution is the *uniform distribution*, which has the same density for each point in a certain interval. If $U \sim \text{Unif}([a, b])$, the density is given by

$$f_U(u) = \begin{cases} \frac{1}{b-a}, & \text{if } a \leq u \leq b, \\ 0, & \text{else.} \end{cases}$$

It is important to understand that the probability density values cannot be interpreted as probabilities. In particular

$$f_X(x) \nleq 1.$$

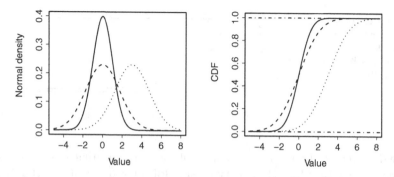

Fig. 1.5 Density functions (*left*) and cumulative distribution functions (*right*) of Norm(μ, σ^2) distribution with parameters (0, 1) (*solid*), (0, 3) (*dashed*), and (3, 3) (*dotted*)

As an easy counterexample, let us consider a uniform random variable U on an interval $[a, b]$. For the interval $[a, b] = [0, 0.5]$, the density function is $f_U(u) = 2$ for each value u inside the interval. Moreover, by moving the right boundary b of the interval towards a, we can make $f_U(u)$ arbitrarily large. Thus, it clearly cannot be interpreted as a probability. The integral of the density over any subinterval is of course still a probability.

1.3 The Normal Distribution

Probably the best known continuous distribution is the *normal distribution*, sometimes also called the *Gaussian distribution*, as it was first completely described by C. F. Gauß. This distribution has two parameters, μ and σ^2. Its probability density function is

$$f(x; \mu, \sigma^2) = \frac{1}{\sqrt{2\pi\sigma^2}} \, e^{-\frac{(x-\mu)^2}{2\sigma^2}} \, .$$

The normal density function has the famous bell-shaped curve and is symmetric around μ; its "width" is determined by σ. Figure 1.5 (left) shows the density of three normal distributions with parameters $(\mu, \sigma^2) = (0, 1)$, $(0, 3)$, and $(3, 3)$, respectively. The corresponding cumulative distribution functions are given in Fig. 1.5 (right).

The normal distribution is so important in probability theory and statistics, that its density and cumulative distribution functions even have their own letters reserved for them: $\phi(x; \mu, \sigma^2)$ for the pdf and $\Phi(x; \mu, \sigma^2)$ for the cdf. If no parameters are given, the two functions refer to the *standard normal distribution* with $\mu = 0$ and $\sigma = 1$.

One of the helpful properties of the normal distribution is that whenever we scale a normal random variable X by multiplying with a fixed a and then shift it by some fixed value b to the new random variable $Y = aX + b$, this new random variable is also normally distributed: with $X \sim$ Norm(μ, σ^2), we have that $Y \sim$

$\text{Norm}(a\mu + b, a^2\sigma^2)$. In particular, for $X \sim \text{Norm}(\mu_X, \sigma_X^2)$,

$$Z = \frac{X - \mu_X}{\sigma_X} \sim \text{Norm}(0, 1)$$

has a standard normal distribution.

Moreover, the sum of random variables with the same, arbitrary distribution does in general not have the same distribution as the variables themselves. In contrast, adding independent normal random variables always leads to a new normal random variable. Let $X_1 \sim \text{Norm}(\mu_1, \sigma_1^2)$ and $X_2 \sim \text{Norm}(\mu_2, \sigma_2^2)$ be two independent normal variables, potentially with different parameters. Then,

$$X_1 + X_2 \sim \text{Norm}(\mu_1 + \mu_2, \sigma_1^2 + \sigma_2^2).$$

1.4 Important Distributions and Their Relations

We will later consider many more distributions that occur in various statistical contexts. In this section, we briefly review some of these and show how they are related among each other. This will later allow us to more easily understand how many distributions of estimators and test statistics are derived.

Arguably the most frequently encountered distributions in statistics are those in the following list:

- Normal distribution, with parameters μ and σ^2,
- Student's t-distribution, with parameter d, the degrees of freedom,
- χ^2-distribution, with parameter d, the degrees of freedom,
- F-distribution, with parameters m, n, two degrees of freedom.

Instead of listing their density functions and properties here, we refer to the fact that they are easily available in any statistics package. In R, their distribution functions are accessible via the functions `pnorm`, `pt`, `pchisq`, and `pf`, respectively, where `p` can be replaced by `d, q, r` to get the density and quantile functions, or a random number generator, respectively.

These distributions are related as follows.

- $X \sim \text{Norm}(\mu, \sigma^2) \Rightarrow \frac{X-\mu}{\sigma} \sim \text{Norm}(0, 1)$.
- $Z_1, \ldots, Z_n \sim \text{Norm}(0, 1) \Rightarrow \sum_{i=1}^{n} Z_i^2 \sim \chi^2(n)$, if the Z_i are independent.
- $X_1 \sim \chi^2(n), X_2 \sim \chi^2(m) \Rightarrow \frac{\frac{1}{n}X_1}{\frac{1}{m}X_2} \sim F(n, m)$, if X_1, X_2 are independent.
- $Z \sim \text{Norm}(0, 1), X \sim \chi^2(n) \Rightarrow \frac{Z}{\sqrt{\frac{1}{n}X}} \sim t(n)$.

- $X \sim t(m) \Rightarrow X^2 \sim F(1, m)$.
- $X_1 \sim \chi^2(n), X_2 \sim \chi^2(m) \Rightarrow X_1 + X_2 \sim \chi^2(n+m)$, if X_1, X_2 are independent.
- $X_n \sim t(n) \Rightarrow \lim_{n \to \infty} X_n \sim \text{Norm}(0, 1)$.

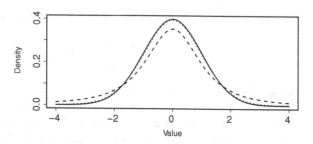

Fig. 1.6 Standard normal density (*solid*) and $t(n)$-densities for $n = 2$ (*dashed*) and $n = 20$ (*dotted*)

As an example, let us consider normally distributed random variables X_i and Y_i with parameters μ_X and μ_Y, respectively, and $\sigma_X = \sigma_Y = 1$. Let us further define the new random variables $V_X = \sum_{i=1}^{n}(X_i - \mu_X)^2$ and $V_Y = \sum_{i=1}^{m}(Y_i - \mu_Y)^2$. These will later be called *variations*, as they measure how "spread out" the values of X and Y are. Both V_X and V_Y are sums of squares of random variables with standard normal distribution. Thus, both V_X and V_Y follow χ^2-distributions with parameters n and m, respectively. Further, their quotient V_X/V_Y is used in regression analysis; we immediately see that it is a quotient of two χ^2-variables and therefore has an $F(n, m)$-distribution if scaled appropriately.

Of particular importance is Student's t-distribution, which is the quotient of a standard normal random variable and a scaled χ^2-variable. For $n - 1$ degrees of freedom, the $t(n - 1)$-distribution has density

$$f(t; n) = \frac{\Gamma\left(\frac{n+1}{2}\right)}{\sqrt{n\pi}\frac{n}{2}\left(1 + \frac{t^2}{n}\right)^{\frac{n+1}{2}}}.$$

The densities of this distribution, with $n = 2$ and $n = 20$ degrees of freedom, are given in Fig. 1.6 together with the standard normal density. With increasing n, the t-distribution approaches the standard normal as claimed, but has substantially heavier tails for few degrees of freedom.

1.5 Quantiles

While the cumulative distribution function $F_X(x)$ describes the probability of a random variable X to take a value below a certain value x, the *quantiles* describe the converse: the α-quantile is the value x such that $F_X(x) = \alpha$, i.e., the value for which the random variable has a probability of α to take that or a lower value. Slight difficulties might arise if there is not an exact value x but a whole interval, but the interpretation remains the same. The *quantile function* is then (neglecting technicalities) given by $F_X^{-1}(\alpha)$, the inverse function of the cdf. Thus, if $\mathbb{P}(X \leq q) = \alpha$, then q is the α-quantile of X.

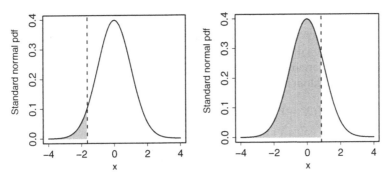

Fig. 1.7 Density of standard normal distribution with 0.05-quantile (*left*) and 0.8-quantile (*right*). The gray areas therefore correspond to probabilities of 0.05 and 0.8, respectively

The 0.05- and the 0.8-quantile of a standard normal distribution are given in Fig. 1.7 (left and right, respectively) as vertical dashed lines. The α-quantile of the standard normal distribution is denoted by z_α, thus $z_{0.05} = \Phi^{-1}(0.05) \approx -1.645$ and $z_{0.8} = \Phi^{-1}(0.8) \approx 0.842$. Using the symmetry of the standard normal distribution, $z_{1-\alpha} = -z_\alpha$.

1.6 Moments

While the distribution of a random variable is completely described by the cumulative distribution function or the density/mass function, it is often helpful to describe its main properties by just a few key numbers. Of particular interest are the *expectation* and the *variance*.

1.6.1 Expectation

The *expectation, expected value,* or *mean* is the number

$$\mathbb{E}(X) := \int_{-\infty}^{\infty} x f(x) dx$$

for a continuous, and

$$\mathbb{E}(X) := \sum_{k=-\infty}^{\infty} k \mathbb{P}(X = k)$$

for a discrete random variable X. The expectation describes the *location* of the distribution, which informally is the center value around which the possible values of X disperse; it is often denoted by the letter μ. The expectation behaves nicely when summing random variables or multiplying them with constants. For random variables X, Y and a non-random number a we have:

$$\mathbb{E}(X + Y) = \mathbb{E}(X) + \mathbb{E}(Y),$$
$$\mathbb{E}(aX) = a\mathbb{E}(X),$$
$$\mathbb{E}(XY) = \mathbb{E}(X)\mathbb{E}(Y) \text{ if X,Y are independent.}$$

1.6.2 Variance and Standard Deviation

The *variance* of a random variable X describes how much its values disperse around the expected value and is a measure for the width of its distribution. It is defined as

$$\text{Var}(X) := \mathbb{E}\big((X - \mathbb{E}(X))^2\big),$$

the mean squared distance of values to the expected value and is often denoted by σ^2. A short calculation gives the alternative description

$$\text{Var}(X) = \mathbb{E}(X^2) - (\mathbb{E}(X))^2.$$

The variance is not linear and we have the following relations for random variables X, Y and non-random numbers a, b:

$$\text{Var}(X + Y) = \text{Var}(X) + \text{Var}(Y) \text{ if X,Y are independent,}$$
$$\text{Var}(X + b) = \text{Var}(X),$$
$$\text{Var}(aX) = a^2\text{Var}(X).$$

The square-root σ is called the *standard deviation*. While it does not contain any more information than the variance, it is often more convenient for applications, as it is easier to interpret and has the same physical units as the random variable itself. It is a measure for the *scale* of a distribution, as rescaling X by any factor a changes the standard deviation by the same factor.

Expectation and variance completely specify a normal distribution, whose two parameters they are. For $X \sim \text{Norm}(\mu, \sigma^2)$, the following approximations are often useful: the probability of X taking a value x at most one standard deviation away from the mean, i.e., $x \in [\mu - \sigma, \mu + \sigma]$, is roughly 70%. Similarly, the probabilities of observing a value at most 2, respectively 3 standard deviations from the mean, are roughly 95% and 99%, respectively. Note that these probabilities can be very different for non-normal random variables.

Fig. 1.8 Gamma (*solid*) and
normal (*dashed*) densities
both with mean $\mu = 4$ and
variance $\sigma^2 = 8$,
corresponding to Gamma
parameters $k = 2$ and $\theta = 2$

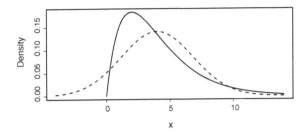

Example **7** For introducing yet another continuous distribution on the go, let us
consider the *Gamma distribution* with shape parameter k and scale parameter θ.
It has density function $f(x; k, \theta) = x^{k-1} \exp(-x/\theta)/\theta^k \Gamma(k)$, is only defined for
$x > 0$, and describes the distribution of the sum of k exponentially distributed
waiting times, each with rate parameter θ (thus the time to wait for the kth event).
This density function is usually not symmetric. For $k = 2$ and $\theta = 2$, the distribution
has expectation $\mu = k\theta = 4$ and variance $\sigma^2 = k\theta^2 = 8$; its density is shown in
Fig. 1.8 (solid line). For comparison, a normal distribution with the same expectation
and variance is plotted by a dashed line. As we can see, the density functions look
very different, although both have the same mean and variance. For additionally
capturing their different shapes, higher moments are needed (see Sect. 1.6.5).

Example **8** Let us consider the following model of a random DNA sequence as introduced earlier: we assume independence among the nucleotides and in each position,
the probabilities of having a particular nucleotide are p_A, p_C, p_G, p_T, respectively.
We investigate two sequences of length n by comparing the nucleotides in the same
position. Assume that the sequences are completely random and unrelated. At any
position, the probability of a match is then $p := p_A^2 + p_C^2 + p_G^2 + p_T^2$, as both
nucleotides have to be the same. Let us set $M_i = 1$ if the sequences match in position i and $M_i = 0$ else.

To decide whether two given sequences are related, we compute the number of
matching nucleotides and compare it to the number of matches we expect just by
chance. If the observed number is much higher than the expected number, we claim
that the sequences are in fact related.[1]

The total number of matches in two random sequences of length n is given by
$M := M_1 + \cdots + M_n$ and follows a binomial distribution: $M \sim \text{Binom}(n, p)$.
Applying the linearity of the expectation and some algebra, we compute the expected
number of matches:

---

[1] As a word of caution for the biological audience: this argument does not hold for *aligned*
sequences, as the alignment maximizes the number of matches, and this maximum has a different
distribution.

$$E(M) = \sum_{k=-\infty}^{\infty} k \mathbb{P}(M = k)$$

$$= \sum_{k=0}^{n} k \binom{n}{k} p^k (1 - p)^{n-k}$$

$$= \sum_{k=1}^{n} np \frac{(n-1)!}{(k-1)!((n-1)-(k-1))!} p^{k-1} (1-p)^{(n-1)-(k-1)}$$

$$= np \sum_{k=1}^{n} \binom{n-1}{k-1} p^{k-1} (1-p)^{(n-1)-(k-1)}$$

$$= np,$$

where the last equality holds because we have the pmf of a Binom $(n-1, p)$ variable in the sum, which sums to one. The result also makes intuitive sense: the expected number of matches is the proportion p of matches times the number of nucleotides n. Consequently, for sequences of length $n = 100$, with nucleotide probabilities all equal to 0.25, the probability of a match is $p = 0.25$ and we expect to see 25 matches just by chance if the sequences are unrelated.

How surprised are we if we observe 29 matches? Would this give us reason to conclude that the sequences might in fact be related? To answer these questions, we would need to know how likely it is to see a deviation of 4 from the expected value. This information is captured by the variance, which we can calculate as

$$\text{Var}(M) = \text{Var}(M_1) + \cdots + \text{Var}(M_n),$$

because we assumed that the nucleotides are independent among positions. Using the definition of the variance,

$$\text{Var}(M_1) = \mathbb{E}((M_1)^2) - (\mathbb{E}(M_1))^2 = (0^2 \times (1-p) + 1^2 \times p) - p^2 = p(1-p),$$

and we immediately get

$$\text{Var}(M) = n \text{Var}(M_1) = np(1 - p) = 18.75$$

and a standard deviation of 4.33 These values indicate that the deviation of the observed number of matches (=29) from the expected number of matches (=25) is within the range that we would expect to see in unrelated sequences, giving no evidence of the sequences being related. We will see in Chap. 3 how these arguments can be used for a more rigorous analysis.

1.6.3 Z-Scores

Using the expectation and variance of any random variable X, we can also compute a normalized version Z with expectation zero and variance one by

$$Z = \frac{X - \mathbb{E}(X)}{\sqrt{\text{Var}(X)}}.$$

This random variable is sometimes called the *Z-score*. For a given realization x of X, the associated value z of Z tells us how many standard deviations σ the value x is away from its expected value. In essence, this rescales to units of one standard deviation.

Importantly, however, the distribution of Z might not belong to the same family as the distribution of X. An important exception is the normal distribution, where $Z \sim \text{Norm}(0, 1)$ if $X \sim \text{Norm}(\mu, \sigma^2)$.

1.6.4 Covariance and Independence

For two random variables X and Y, we can compute the *covariance*

$$\text{Cov}(X, Y) = \mathbb{E}\left((X - \mathbb{E}(X))(Y - \mathbb{E}(Y))\right),$$

to measure how much the variable X varies together with the variable Y (and vice-versa). With this information, we can also calculate the variance of dependent variables by

$$\text{Var}(X + Y) = \text{Var}(X) + \text{Var}(Y) + 2\text{Cov}(X, Y).$$

As a special case, $\text{Cov}(X, X) = \text{Var}(X)$. For independent X and Y, the covariance is zero. The converse, however, is *not* true, as the following counterexample demonstrates.

Example 9 Let us consider possible outcomes $\Omega = \{1, 2, 3, 4\}$ and a probability measure given by $\mathbb{P}(\{1\}) = \mathbb{P}(\{2\}) = \frac{2}{5}$ and $\mathbb{P}(\{3\}) = \mathbb{P}(\{4\}) = \frac{1}{10}$. Let us further define the two random variables X and Y by

ω	1	2	3	4
X	1	-1	2	-2
Y	-1	1	2	-2

These two random variables are completely dependent. A simple calculation gives the expectations:

$$\mathbb{E}(X) = \sum_{k=1}^{4} k\mathbb{P}(X = k) = 1 \times \frac{2}{5} + (-1) \times \frac{2}{5} + 2 \times \frac{1}{10} + (-2) \times \frac{1}{10}$$

$$= 0,$$

$$\mathbb{E}(Y) = 0.$$

From this, we calculate the covariance of the two variables as

$$
\begin{aligned}
\mathrm{Cov}(X, Y) &= \mathbb{E}(XY) - \mathbb{E}(X)\mathbb{E}(Y) \\
&= (-1) \times \frac{2}{5} + (-1) \times \frac{2}{5} + 4 \times \frac{1}{10} + 4 \times \frac{1}{10} - 0 \times 0 \\
&= 0.
\end{aligned}
$$

Thus, although the covariance of the two random variables is zero, they are nevertheless completely dependent.

Another derived measure for the dependency is the *correlation coefficient* of X and Y, given by

$$
R = \frac{\mathrm{Cov}(X, Y)}{\sqrt{\mathrm{Var}(X)}\sqrt{\mathrm{Var}(Y)}}.
$$

The correlation is also often denoted $\rho(X, Y)$ and takes values in $[-1, 1]$, where $R = \pm 1$ indicates very strong dependence. Even then, however, this does not mean that either X or Y cause each other. As an example, the correlation to see a wet street and people carrying an umbrella is likely to be very strong. But carrying an umbrella clearly does not cause the street to be wet. In fact, both are likely caused simultaneously by rainfall, a third variable that was not accounted for. Thus, *correlation is not causation.*

1.6.5 General Moments; Skewness and Kurtosis

The *kth (central) moments* are given by

$$
\mathbb{E}\left((X)^k\right) \quad \text{and} \quad \mathbb{E}\left((X - \mathbb{E}(X))^k\right) \quad \text{respectively;}
$$

the variance is recovered as the second central moment.

The third central moment, normalized by the standard deviation, is called the *skewness* and describes how symmetric the values spread around the mean by

$$
\mathrm{skew}(X) = \mathbb{E}\left(\left(\frac{X - \mathbb{E}(X)}{\sqrt{\mathrm{Var}(X)}}\right)^3\right).
$$

A negative skewness indicates that the distribution "leans" towards the left and a perfectly symmetric distribution has skewness zero.

The (normalized) fourth central moment is called the *kurtosis* and describes how fast the density function approaches zero in the left and right tail by

$$
\mathrm{kurtosis}(X) = \mathbb{E}\left(\left(\frac{X - \mathbb{E}(X)}{\sqrt{\mathrm{Var}(X)}}\right)^4\right) - 3.
$$

A negative kurtosis indicates that the variance is mostly caused by many values moderately far away from the mean, whereas a positive kurtosis indicates that the variance is determined by few extreme deviations from the mean. The sole reason for subtracting 3 is to make the kurtosis equal to zero for a normal distribution.

For the above Gamma-distribution with shape parameter $k = 2$ and scale parameter $\theta = 2$ (cf. Fig. 1.8), we compute a skewness of 1.414 and a kurtosis of 3. Together with the expectation and the variance, these numbers often already give a reasonable description of the shape of the density function.

1.7 Important Limit Theorems

The sum of many similar random variables is of particular interest in many applications. In this section, we will discuss two important limit theorems that allow us to compute its distribution in a variety of situations and explain the omnipresence of the normal distribution in applications.

The first theorem gives the *Law of Large Numbers (LLN)*. Consider a random sample $X_1, \ldots, X_n$, described by n random variables. We assume that each random variable has the same distribution, and all are independent from each other, a property called *independent and identically distributed (iid)*. In particular, they all have the same expectation $\mathbb{E}(X_1) = \cdots = \mathbb{E}(X_n)$. The theorem then says that if we take their arithmetic mean $\bar{X}$, it approaches the expectation as we increase n:

$$\bar{X} = \frac{X_1 + \cdots + X_n}{n} \to \mathbb{E}(X_1) \text{ as } n \to \infty.$$

This theorem thus gives one reason why expectation and arithmetic mean are so tightly linked in statistics. Importantly, the theorem does not require the X_i to have any particular distribution.

The second theorem is the *Central Limit Theorem (CLT)*, which gives the reason for the omnipresence of the normal distribution. In essence, it tells us that if we sum up iid random variables, the sum itself will eventually become a random variable with a normal distribution, no matter what was the distribution of the individual random variables. Let us again assume iid random variables X_i, having any distribution with expectation μ and variance σ^2. Then,

$$\frac{\sum_{i=1}^{n} X_i - n\mu}{\sqrt{n}\sigma} \to \text{Norm}(0, 1) \text{ as } n \to \infty,$$

or, equivalently,

$$\sqrt{n}\frac{\bar{X} - \mu}{\sigma} \to \text{Norm}(0, 1) \text{ as } n \to \infty.$$

1.8 Visualizing Distributions

Given a random sample drawn from a distribution, it is often helpful to visualize this data and some of its properties like the mean and variance. Plotting the sample points together with a given theoretical distribution often provides enough information to decide whether the distribution "fits" the data or not, i.e., if the data might have been drawn from this distribution. Such *descriptive statistics* are a large topic in themselves, and we will only present some examples that are helpful in later chapters.

1.8.1 Summaries

A first impression of a given set of data is given by simply stating some of the key moments and quantiles of the data. In R, these are directly computed using the summary() function. For 50 sample points from a normal distribution with parameters $\mu = 10$ and $\sigma^2 = 6$, we get the following output:

```
Min. 1st Qu. Median  Mean 3rd Qu.  Max.
5.137  8.795   9.953 10.070 11.220 15.030
```

In this summary, the minimal and maximal values are given together with the expected value and the 0.25-quantile (1st quartile), the 0.5-quantile (called the *median* and the 2nd quartile), and the 0.75-quantile (3rd quartile).

Similarly, for 50 samples from an exponential distribution with parameter $\lambda = 0.4$:

```
Min.   1st Qu. Median   Mean 3rd Qu.   Max.
0.06219 0.60800 1.29100 2.54000 3.14100 19.09000
```

These summaries already reflect the symmetry of the normal data around their mean and the skewness of the exponential, which has most of its sample points at small values, but also contains comparably few large values.

1.8.2 Plotting Empirical Distributions

Let us assume that we gathered some data and assume it follows a normal distribution. Plotting the empirical and the theoretical density or cumulative distribution functions then gives a first impression whether this might be true. For example, Fig. 1.9 gives these functions for $n = 50$ normal samples $X_i \sim \text{Norm}(10, 6)$.

The *empirical density function* of the data is estimated by summing "smeared out" versions of the sample points, such as by assuming a Gaussian bell-curve over each point and summing up the individual values of all these curves. The *empirical cumulative distribution function (ecdf)* is computed by the function

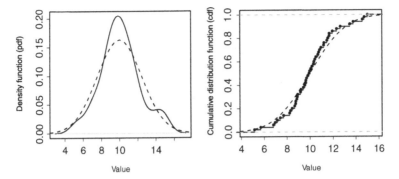

Fig. 1.9 Empirical (*solid*) and theoretical (*dashed*) density functions (*left*) and cumulative distribution functions (*right*) of 50 Norm(10, 6) sample points

$$\hat{F}_n(x) = \frac{H_n(x)}{n},$$

where $H_n(x)$ is the number of sample points smaller than x. This leads to a step function, which in the example quite closely follows the theoretical function.

In practice, the similarity of the empirical and theoretical densities or cumulative distribution functions is often very difficult to judge by eye.

1.8.3 Quantile–Quantile Plots

Another way of comparing two distributions is by plotting their quantile functions. This is extremely helpful when plotting the theoretical quantiles of an assumed distribution against the empirical quantiles of some data. For this, all parameters of the theoretical distribution have to be specified.

An important exception is the normal distribution, which can be compared to samples without knowing its parameter values. Here is how this works: we sort the data $x_1, \ldots, x_n$ such that $x_{(1)} \leq \cdots \leq x_{(n)}$ and thus $x_{(i)}$ is the ith smallest value of the dataset, which is the best guess for the $\frac{i}{n}$-quantile of the distribution. If the data actually stem from a normal distribution with some unknown parameters μ and σ^2, the quantiles relate by

$$x_{(i)} \approx \mu + \sigma \times z_{i/n},$$

where $z_{i/n}$ is the theoretical i/n-quantile of the standard normal distribution. Regardless of the actual parameter values, this is the equation of a line with slope σ and intercept μ. If we therefore plot the points

$$\left(x_{(i)}, z_{i/n} \right),$$

we expect to see a straight line, regardless of the values of μ and σ^2.

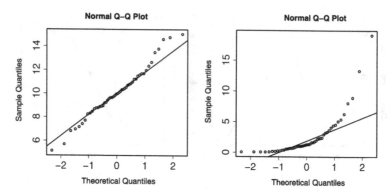

Fig. 1.10 Normal quantile–quantile plot of 50 Norm(10, 6) sample points (*left*) and 50 Exp(0.4) points (*right*). The solid line denotes the theoretical quantile of a normal distribution. While the normal data fit the line nicely, the exponential data deviate strongly from the expected quantiles of a normal distribution

A quantile-quantile plot for a normal sample is given in Fig. 1.10 (left) together with the theoretical quantiles (solid line). For comparison, sample points from an exponential distribution are plotted together with the normal distribution quantiles in Fig. 1.10 (right). As we can see, the agreement of the theoretical and the empirical quantiles is quite good for the normal sample, but it is poor for the exponential sample, especially in the tails.

Quantile plots can be generated in R using the function qqplot(). The functions qqnorm() and qqline() allow comparison to the normal distribution.

1.8.4 Barplots and Boxplots

It is still very popular to give data in terms of a bar with the height corresponding to the expectation and an additional error bar on top to indicate the standard deviation. However, this only shows two key numbers of the whole data (expectation and standard deviation), and does not allow to see how the data actually distribute. A much more informative alternative to plot data is to use the *boxplot*. It shows several parameters simultaneously: a rectangle denotes the positions of the 0.25- and 0.75-quantiles, with a horizontal line in the box showing the median (0.5-quantile). Thus, the middle 50% of the data are contained in that rectangle. On the top and bottom of the rectangle, the "whiskers" show the range of 1.5 times the distance between the 0.25- and 0.75-quantiles. Sample points outside this range are plotted individually. The previous normal and exponential data are both normalized to mean 2 and standard deviation 1 and the resulting data are shown as a barplot (left) and boxplot (right) in Fig. 1.11. In the barplot, no difference between the two samples can be noticed, while the different distributions of the data, the skewness of the exponential, and the symmetry of the normal are immediately recognized in the boxplot. Barplots with

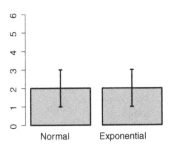 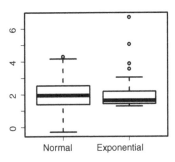

Fig. 1.11 Barplots (*left*) and boxplots (*right*) of normal and exponential data, both with mean 2 and standard deviation 1. Left: Barplots show no difference in the data, with both samples having mean 2 given by the height of the bar and standard deviation 1 indicated by the error bars. Right: Boxplots show the 0.25- and 0.75-quantiles, as the bottom and top of the box, respectively, and the median as a horizontal line. Whiskers denote the range of 1.5 times the dispersion of the 0.25- to the 0.75-quantile, sample points further away are given as individual points. The different distributions of the samples can clearly be seen

out error bars and boxplots can be generated in R using the functions `barplot()` and `boxplot()`, respectively.

1.9 Summary

Probability theory allows us to study the properties of non-deterministic quantities. By defining a probability measure, we can compute the probability of events and their combinations.

A random variable's distribution is given by its cumulative distribution function and the probability mass function for discrete and the density function for continuous random variables. Importantly, the density $f_X(x)$ is not a probability. For a distribution of a random variable X, we can compute the α-quantile as the value q_α such that $\mathbb{P}(X \leq q_\alpha) = \alpha$.

Important discrete distributions are the Binomial and geometric distribution, important continuous distributions are the normal distribution, the exponential, and various statistical distributions, including the t-, F-, and χ^2-distributions, which are all related.

Several interesting properties of a probability distribution are given by its moments, some of which are the expectation, describing the location, the variance, describing the scale and the skewness and kurtosis, describing the asymmetry and heaviness of the tails, respectively.

We can visualize empirical distributions of given random samples using various graphs, such as bar- and box-plots and the quantile-quantile plot. The latter also allows us to easily assess if a given random sample is normally distributed.

Chapter 2
Estimation

Abstract Estimation is the inference of properties of a distribution from an observed random sample. Estimators can be derived by various approaches. To quantify the quality of a given estimate, confidence intervals can be computed; the bootstrap is a general purpose method for this. Vulnerability of some estimators to sample contaminations leads to robust alternatives.

Keywords Maximum-likelihood · Confidence interval · Bootstrap

> *"Data! Data! Data!" he cried impatiently. "I can't make bricks without clay"*
>
> Sherlock Holmes

2.1 Introduction

We assume that n independent and identically distributed random samples $X_1, \ldots, X_n$ are drawn, whose realizations form an observation $x_1, \ldots, x_n$. Our goal is to infer one or more parameters θ of the distribution of the X_i. For this, we construct an *estimator* $\hat{\theta}_n$ by finding a function g, such that

$$\hat{\theta}_n = g(X_1, \ldots, X_n)$$

is a "good guess" of the true value θ. Since $\hat{\theta}_n$ depends on the data, it is a random variable. Finding its distribution allows us to compute confidence intervals that quantify how likely it is that the true value θ is close to the estimate $\hat{\theta}_n$.

Example 10 Let us revisit the problem of sequence matching from Example 8 (p. 19) we already know that the number of matches in two random sequences is a random variable $M \sim$ Binom (n, p), but do not know the probability p, and want to infer it from given data. For this, let us assume we are given two sequences of length n each, and record the matches $m_1, \ldots, m_n$, where again $m_i = 1$ if position i is a match, and $m_i = 0$ if it is a mismatch, as well as the total number of matches $m = m_1 + \cdots + m_n$.

H.-M. Kaltenbach, *A Concise Guide to Statistics*, SpringerBriefs in Statistics, DOI: 10.1007/978-3-642-23502-3_2, © Hans-Michael Kaltenbach 2012

For any fixed value of p, we can compute the probability to see exactly the observed matches $m_1, \ldots, m_n$. The main new idea is to consider this probability as a function of the parameter p for given observations. This function is known as the *likelihood function*

$$L_n(p) = \mathbb{P}(M_1 = m_1, \ldots, M_n = m_n) = \prod_{i=1}^{n} \mathbb{P}(M_i = m_i) = p^m (1 - p)^{n-m};$$

note that we can only write the joint probability as a product because we assume the positions (and therefore the individual matches) to be independent. We then seek the value $\hat{p}_n$ that maximizes this likelihood and gives the highest probability for the observed outcome. In this sense, it therefore "best" explains the observed data. Maximizing the likelihood is straightforward in this case: we differentiate the likelihood function with respect to p and find its roots by solving the equation

$$\frac{\partial L_n(p)}{\partial p} = 0.$$

Taking the derivative of $L_n(p)$ requires repeated application of the product-rule. It is therefore more convenient to use the *log-likelihood* for the maximization, given by

$$\ell_n(p) = \log L_n(p) = \sum_{i=1}^{n} \log \mathbb{P}(M_i = m_i) = m \log(p) + (n - m) \log(1 - p).$$

Maximizing either $L_n(p)$ or $\ell_n(p)$ yields the exact same result, as the logarithm is a strictly increasing function, but we can conveniently differentiate each summand individually in the log-likelihood. In our case,

$$0 = \frac{\partial \ell_n(p)}{\partial p} = m \frac{1}{p} + (n - m) \left(-\frac{1}{1 - p} \right),$$

which gives

$$\frac{m}{p} = \frac{n - m}{1 - p} \iff p = \frac{m}{n}.$$

Thus, the desired estimate of the parameter value p is $\hat{p}_n = m/n$, the proportion of matches in the sequence.

It is important to understand the fundamental difference between the parameter p and its estimate $\hat{p}_n$: the parameter p is a fixed number, relating to the model describing the experiment. It is independent of the particular outcome m of the experiment. In contrast, its estimate $\hat{p}_n$ is a function of the data and takes different values for different samples. For studying general properties of this estimator, we will therefore consider $\hat{p}_n$ as the random variable M/n rather than its realization m/n. It then has

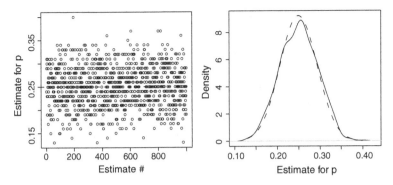

Fig. 2.1 *Left*: values of 1000 repetitions of estimating the matching probability of Binom(100,0.25) experiments. *Right*: density of estimate (*solid*) and Norm(0.25,0.001875) approximation (*dashed*)

a distribution and if we were to repeat the same experiment over and over, p would always be the same, but the estimate would yield a different realization of $\hat{p}_n$ each time.

Because an estimator is a random variable, it is helpful to either compute its entire distribution or some of its moments. For our example, we can easily work out the expectation and the variance of our estimator:

$$\mathbb{E}(\hat{p}_n) = \mathbb{E}\left(\frac{M}{n}\right) = \frac{1}{n}\mathbb{E}(M) = \frac{np}{n} = p,$$

which shows that the estimator is *unbiased* and thus—on average—yields the correct value for the parameter, and

$$\mathrm{Var}(\hat{p}_n) = \frac{1}{n^2}\mathrm{Var}(M) = \frac{p(1-p)}{n}.$$

The variance of the estimator decreases with increasing sample size n, which is intuitively plausible: by using more data, we are more confident about the correct value of the parameter p and expect the estimator to get closer to the true value with high probability. We also get a lower variance of the estimate if the variance of the data is smaller.

The estimator of a true parameter value $p = 0.25$ is studied in Fig. 2.1 on 1000 pairs of unrelated sequences of length 100. On the left, the values of $\hat{p}_n$ are given for each such pair. Most estimates lie reasonably close to the true value, but there are also some larger deviations. On the right, the empirical density function of $\hat{p}_n$ is given (solid line) together with a normal density with the same expectation and variance (dashed line). The values of the estimate closely follow the normal distribution and the mean nicely corresponds to the correct parameter value p.

2.2 Constructing Estimators

To derive an estimator for a parameter θ, we need to construct the function $g(X_1, \ldots, X_n)$. There are multiple methods to do this and we will discuss the maximum-likelihood and the least-squares approach in more depth. Both methods rely on finding the parameter value that "best" explains the observed data, but there definition of "best" is different and requires finding the minimum or maximum of a certain function. A third approach, the minimax principle, will be presented in a more general framework in Sect. 2.5.

2.2.1 Maximum-Likelihood

To apply maximum-likelihood estimation in the general case, we need to specify a *family of distributions* that is parametrized by θ such that each value of θ selects one particular distribution from this family. In the previous example, this family was the set of all binomial distributions with fixed n, where each value for p selects one particular member of this family.

Here, we consider the density function $f(x; \theta)$, describing the family of distributions, and aim at estimating the parameter θ. The *likelihood function* for this parameter is

$$L_n(\theta) = \prod_{i=1}^{n} f(x_i; \theta),$$

which in the discrete case corresponds to the joint probability that the underlying distribution generates the observed sample $x_1, \ldots, x_n$. For a family of continuous distributions, this product can no longer be directly interpreted as a probability, but the overall reasoning remains the same. The corresponding *log-likelihood function* is

$$\ell_n(\theta) = \log(L_n(\theta)) = \sum_{i=1}^{n} \log(f(x_i; \theta)).$$

The *maximum-likelihood estimator (MLE)* $\hat{\theta}_n$ of θ then corresponds to the value that maximizes the likelihood functions:

$$\hat{\theta}_n := \mathrm{argmax}_\theta L_n(\theta) = \mathrm{argmax}_\theta \ell_n(\theta).$$

Example 11 Let us suppose that we perform n measurements and have good reason to expect them to be normally distributed such that $X_1, \ldots, X_n \sim \mathrm{Norm}(\mu, \sigma^2)$. The normal distribution can often be justified with the Central Limit Theorem. We want to estimate both parameters from the n observed values $x_1, \ldots, x_n$ using the maximum-likelihood approach. Let us denote the parameters as $\theta = (\mu, \sigma)$ and start with setting up the likelihood function

$$L_n(\theta) = \frac{1}{\pi} \prod_{i=1}^{n} \frac{1}{\sigma} \exp\left(-\frac{(X_i - \mu)^2}{2\sigma^2}\right) \propto \sigma^{-n} \exp\left(-\frac{1}{2\sigma^2} \sum_{i=1}^{n} (X_i - \mu)^2\right),$$

where we ignored constant factors in the second equation, as they do not contribute to the maximization (the symbol $\propto$ means "proportional to"). Abbreviating $\bar{X} = \frac{1}{n} \sum X_i$ and $S^2 = \frac{1}{n} \sum (X_i - \bar{X})^2$, we can eliminate the sum and simplify to

$$L_n(\theta) \propto \sigma^{-n} \exp\left(-\frac{nS^2}{2\sigma^2}\right) \exp\left(-\frac{n(\bar{X} - \mu)^2}{2\sigma^2}\right),$$

from which we immediately derive the log-likelihood function

$$\ell_n(\theta) \propto -n \log(\sigma) - \frac{nS^2}{2\sigma^2} - \frac{n(\bar{X} - \mu)^2}{2\sigma^2}.$$

We maximize this function by taking the derivatives with respect to μ and σ, respectively. For deriving $\hat{\mu}_n$, the equation reads

$$\frac{\partial \ell_n(\theta)}{\partial \mu} = -\frac{n}{2\sigma^2} \left(-2\bar{X} + 2\mu\right),$$

and finding the roots yields the estimator

$$-2\bar{X} + 2\mu = 0 \iff \bar{X} = \mu.$$

Not surprising, the arithmetic mean is an estimator for the expectation. The maximum-likelihood estimators for the two parameters are then

$$\hat{\mu}_n = \bar{X} = \frac{1}{n} \sum_{i=1}^{n} X_i \quad \text{and} \quad \hat{\sigma}_n^2 = S^2 = \frac{1}{n} \sum_{i=1}^{n} (X_i - \bar{X})^2,$$

where the derivation of $\hat{\sigma}_n$ follows the same ideas.

Calculating the distribution of an estimator will become crucial for establishing the bounds of a particular estimate. While this calculation is often difficult for general estimators, maximum-likelihood estimators have the convenient property of being *asymptotically normal*. Formally,

$$\frac{\hat{\theta}_n - \theta}{\sqrt{Var(\hat{\theta}_n)}} \rightarrow \text{Norm}(0, 1) \text{ as } n \rightarrow \infty,$$

which simply means that if the sample size gets large enough, *any* maximum-likelihood estimator has a normal distribution. In retrospect, this explains the surprisingly good fit of the empirical and normal density in our introductory example (see Fig. 2.1 (right)).

2.2.2 Least-Squares

Instead of maximizing the likelihood of the observed outcome, we can also construct an estimator by looking at the distance of the observed outcome and the outcome that we would expect with a particular parameter value. The value that minimizes this distance is then an estimate for the parameter.

Let us denote by $h(\theta)$ the expected value of observations for parameter value θ. With measurements x_i, we then minimize the distance

$$d(\theta) = \sum_{i=1}^{n}(x_i - h(\theta))^2.$$

The *least-squares estimate (LSE)* $\hat{\theta}_n$ is then the value that minimized this squared difference between observed and expected data. This is a very common approach in regression (Chap. 4).

Example 12 Let us consider the sequence matching again, this time from a least-squares perspective, and compare the matches with their expected value. At each position i, the expected value of a match is $\mathbb{E}(M_i) = p$, while the observed match m_i is either zero or one. We minimize the sum of their squared differences:

$$\tilde{p}_n = \text{argmin}_p \sum_{i=1}^{n}(m_i - p)^2.$$

Minimization is again done by finding the roots of the derivative. A quick calculation reveals

$$\frac{\partial}{\partial p}\sum_{i=1}^{n}(m_i - p)^2 = \frac{\partial}{\partial p}\left(\sum_{i=1}^{n}m_i^2 - 2p\sum_{i=1}^{n}m_i + \sum_{i=1}^{n}p^2\right) = 0 - 2m + 2np,$$

which yields $\tilde{p}_n = \frac{m}{n}$. In this example, the least-squares and the maximum-likelihood estimator are identical, but this is not always the case.

2.2.3 Properties of Estimators

In principle, there is no reason why we should not define an estimator $\hat{\theta}_n = g(X_1, \ldots, X_n) = 0$, which completely ignores the data. It is a formally valid estimator, but quite useless in practice. The question therefore arises, how we can capture properties of an estimator and conclude that, for example the MLE is more useful than the proposed "zero-estimator"?

Consistency. The first useful property of an estimator is *consistency*, which means that with increasing sample size, the estimate approaches the true parameter value:

$$\hat{\theta}_n \to \theta \text{ as } n \to \infty.$$

While all three estimators ($\hat{p}_n$, $\bar{X}$, S^2) in the binomial and normal examples are consistent, the above estimator $\hat{\theta}_n \equiv 0$ is obviously not, because the estimate does not get any closer to the true value, no matter how many samples we take.

Unbiasedness. Even if an estimator is consistent, it might still be that it systematically over- or underestimates the true value and introduces a *bias* in the estimate. The bias is given by the difference of expected and true value

$$\mathbb{E}(\hat{\theta}_n) - \theta,$$

and an estimator is called *unbiased* if this difference is zero. If we were to repeat the same sampling procedure multiple times, an unbiased estimator would on average neither over- nor underestimate the true parameter value.

The following example shows the bias in one of the estimators we constructed earlier.

Example 13 Consider the estimates for the parameters μ and σ^2 of a normal distribution as given above. Are they unbiased? Let us start with $\bar{X}$; its unbiasedness is easily established by exploiting the linearity of the expectation:

$$\mathbb{E}(\bar{X}) = \mathbb{E}\left(\frac{1}{n}\sum_{i=1}^{n} X_i\right) = \frac{1}{n}\sum_{i=1}^{n}\mathbb{E}(X_i) = \frac{1}{n}n\mu = \mu.$$

The calculation for S^2 is slightly more elaborate and we skip some details:

$$\mathbb{E}(S^2) = \frac{1}{n}\sum_{i=1}^{n}\mathbb{E}\left((X_i - \bar{X})^2\right) = \frac{1}{n}\sum_{i=1}^{n}\mathbb{E}\left((X_i - \mu)(\bar{X} - \mu)\right)$$

$$= \sigma^2 - \frac{2}{n}\sigma^2 + \frac{n\sigma^2}{n^2} = \sigma^2\left(1 - \frac{1}{n}\right) \neq \sigma^2.$$

The MLE for the variance is therefore biased and systematically underestimates the true variance. It is nevertheless consistent, as the bias is proportional to $1/n$ and decreases rapidly to zero for increasing n.

The reason for this can presumably be best explained with the following argument: we use n sample points $X_1, \ldots, X_n$ for estimation and thus divide by n. However, we also use the *estimate* $\bar{x}$ instead of the true expectation μ. The value of any sample point is completely determined if we know $\bar{X}$ and the other remaining points. The *degrees of freedom* in the estimate are therefore $n - 1$ rather than n, as we already "used" one degree for estimating μ. Indeed,

$$S^2 = \hat{\sigma}_n^2 = \frac{1}{n-1}\sum_{i=1}^{n}(X_i - \bar{X})^2$$

is an unbiased estimator for the variance, but not a maximum-likelihood estimator.

Properties of ML-Estimators. Conveniently, maximum-likelihood estimators automatically have many desired properties. They are

- *consistent*: they approach the true parameter value with increasing sample size,
- *equivariant*: if r is a function, then $r(\hat{\theta}_n)$ is also the MLE of $r(\theta)$,
- *not* necessarily unbiased, so we need to take caution here,
- *asymptotically normal*: $\dfrac{\hat{\theta}_n - \theta}{\sqrt{\text{Var}(\hat{\theta}_n)}} \rightarrow$ Norm $(0, 1)$ as $n \rightarrow \infty$.

2.3   Confidence Intervals

The discussed properties of estimators provide valuable information for comparing and choosing an estimator, but they say rather little about the quality of a particular estimate. For example, consistency guarantees that the estimated value will approach the true value in the limit, but does not give information on how close it is to the true value, given some data with a certain number of samples.

For quantifying the quality of a particular estimate, we can compute a *confidence interval (CI)* around the estimate $\hat{\theta}_n$, such that this interval covers the true value θ with some high probability $1 - \alpha$. The narrower this interval, the closer we are to the true value, with high probability.

Let us go through the main ideas first, before we look into two concrete examples. For an estimator $\hat{\theta}_n$, the $(1 - \alpha)$-confidence interval is the interval

$$C = \left[\hat{\theta}_n - l, \hat{\theta}_n + u \right],$$

for a lower value l and an upper value u such that

$$\mathbb{P}(\theta \in C) = 1 - \alpha. \tag{2.1}$$

This interval C is random, because the value of $\hat{\theta}_n$ depends on the data. The location of the interval is determined by $\hat{\theta}_n$, and its width depends on the distribution of the estimator and in particular on the estimator's variance $\text{Var}(\hat{\theta}_n)$. If the estimator's variance decreases, the confidence interval gets narrower. This allows us to conclude that the difference of true value and estimate gets smaller with decreasing variance, with high probability. We usually need to work with the square-root of the estimator's variance, which we call the *standard error*:

$$\text{se}(\hat{\theta}_n) = \sqrt{\text{Var}(\hat{\theta}_n)}.$$

For computing the confidence interval, we start by normalizing the estimator by shifting it by (the unknown) true parameter θ and scaling by $1/\text{se}(\hat{\theta}_n)$. Provided the estimator is unbiased, this normalization simply shifts the estimator's distribution by its mean and scales by the standard error, which results in a new random variable with mean zero and standard error one. Equation 2.1 then becomes

$$\mathbb{P}\left(\frac{\hat{\theta}_n - \theta}{\text{se}(\hat{\theta}_n)} \in \left[\frac{-l}{\text{se}(\hat{\theta}_n)}, \frac{u}{\text{se}(\hat{\theta}_n)}\right]\right) = 1 - \alpha. \qquad (2.2)$$

Solving (2.2) requires that we find the two quantiles $q_{\alpha/2}, q_{1-\alpha/2}$ of the distribution of the normalized estimator, with $1 - \alpha/2 - \alpha/2 = 1 - \alpha$. From these quantiles, we work out the upper value $u = q_{1-\alpha/2}\text{se}(\hat{\theta}_n)$ and thus the interval bound $\hat{\theta}_n + q_{1-\alpha/2}\text{se}(\hat{\theta}_n)$, and similar for the lower value l. For an unbiased estimator, the $(1 - \alpha)$-confidence interval therefore takes the general form

$$C = \left[\hat{\theta}_n + q_{\alpha/2}\text{se}(\hat{\theta}_n), \hat{\theta}_n + q_{1-\alpha/2}\text{se}(\hat{\theta}_n)\right],$$

which simplifies by $q_{\alpha/2} = -q_{1-\alpha/2}$ if the estimator additionally has a symmetric distribution around its mean. The two main remaining problems are then to establish the distribution of $\hat{\theta}_n$ to calculate the quantiles and to estimate its variance.

If $\hat{\theta}_n$ is an unbiased maximum-likelihood estimator, we already know that the estimator has a normal distribution and the correct quantiles are $z_{\alpha/2}$ and $z_{1-\alpha/2}$. The shifted and scaled interval is then symmetric around zero and the confidence interval is immediately given by

$$C = \left[\hat{\theta}_n - z_{1-\alpha/2}\text{se}(\hat{\theta}_n), \hat{\theta}_n + z_{1-\alpha/2}\text{se}(\hat{\theta}_n)\right].$$

Before we deal with the more general case of estimators that are not ML, let us first look into two concrete examples and work out confidence intervals for the sequence matching problem and the estimates for the normal parameters.

Example 14 We would like to compute an interval $[\hat{p}_n - l, \hat{p}_n + u]$ around the estimate $\hat{p}_n$ of the matching probability, such that the interval contains the true value p with given probability $1 - \alpha$:

$$\mathbb{P}(p \in [\hat{p}_n - l, \hat{p}_n + u]) = \mathbb{P}(\hat{p}_n - l \le p \le \hat{p}_n + u) = 1 - \alpha.$$

Because $\hat{p}_n$ is the maximum-likelihood estimator of p, its distribution approaches a normal distribution for large n. Its normalized form has a standard normal distribution:

$$\frac{p - \hat{p}_n}{\text{se}(\hat{p}_n)} \sim \text{Norm}(0, 1).$$

We can therefore immediately solve the following equation by using the corresponding quantiles z_α for u and l

$$\mathbb{P}\left(\frac{-l}{\text{se}(\hat{p}_n)} \le \frac{p - \hat{p}_n}{\text{se}(\hat{p}_n)} \le \frac{u}{\text{se}(\hat{p}_n)}\right) = 1 - \alpha.$$

By exploiting the symmetry of the normal distribution, we derive

$$\frac{u}{\text{se}(\hat{p}_n)} = z_{1-\alpha/2} \iff u = z_{1-\alpha/2}\text{se}(\hat{p}_n) \text{ and } l = z_{\alpha/2}\text{se}(\hat{p}_n),$$

The standard error of $\hat{p}_n$ is $\text{se}(\hat{p}_n) = \sqrt{p(1-p)/n}$, leading to the requested confidence interval

$$C = \left[\hat{p}_n + z_{\alpha/2}\sqrt{\frac{\hat{p}_n(1-\hat{p}_n)}{n}}, \, \hat{p}_n + z_{1-\alpha/2}\sqrt{\frac{\hat{p}_n(1-\hat{p}_n)}{n}} \right],$$

where we replaced the unknown true parameter value p by its estimate $\hat{p}_n$.

An immediate caveat of the approximation of the true distribution of the estimator $\hat{p}_n$ by its asymptotic normal distribution is that this confidence interval is only valid for large sample sizes n and parameter values not too close to zero or one. For small p, for example, the confidence interval would also consider the case that $\hat{p}_n$ takes on a negative value, which is not possible. Hence, the approximations for this confidence interval are not always valid and more sophisticated intervals exist.

Example 15 Let us consider the estimator for the expectation of normally distributed data, i.e., $\bar{X} = \frac{1}{n}\sum_{i=1}^{n} X_i$ with $X_i \sim \text{Norm}(\mu, \sigma^2)$. Being the ML-estimator, this random variable has a normal distribution. We already checked that it is unbiased, and we easily compute its variance $\text{Var}(\bar{X})$ as

$$\text{Var}(\bar{X}) = \text{Var}\left(\frac{1}{n}\sum_{i=1}^{n} X_i\right) = \frac{1}{n^2}\sum_{i=1}^{n}\text{Var}(X_i) = \frac{1}{n^2}n\sigma^2 = \frac{\sigma^2}{n},$$

where we could take the sum outside the variance because we assumed the X_i to be independent. Thus, the normalized distribution of the difference in true and estimated mean is

$$\frac{\bar{X} - \mu}{\sigma/\sqrt{n}} \sim \text{Norm}(0, 1).$$

Again, we do not know the true variance and need to estimate is using the unbiased estimator $S^2 = \frac{1}{n-1}\sum_{i=1}^{n}(X_i - \bar{X})^2$, which leads to the normalized random variable

$$\frac{\bar{X} - \mu}{S/\sqrt{n}},$$

which does *not* have a standard normal distribution. We can derive its correct distribution by looking at the estimated variance in more detail. In particular, let us consider the quotient of the true and estimated variance:

$$(n-1)\frac{S^2}{\sigma^2} = (n-1)\frac{\frac{1}{n-1}\sum_{i=1}^{n}(X_i - \bar{X})^2}{\sigma^2} = \sum_{i=1}^{n}\left(\frac{X_i - \bar{X}}{\sigma}\right)^2.$$

Each summand is the square of a standard normal variable and there are $(n-1)$ independent such variables. Thus, from Sect. 1.4, we know that the sum has a χ^2-distribution with $(n-1)$ degrees of freedom. Replacing the true variance by its estimate, we derive the distribution

$$\frac{\bar{X}-\mu}{S/\sqrt{n}} = \frac{\bar{X}-\mu}{\sigma/\sqrt{n}} \times \frac{\sigma/\sqrt{n}}{S/\sqrt{n}} \sim \frac{\text{Norm}(0,1)}{\sqrt{\frac{1}{n-1}\chi^2(n-1)}},$$

which from Sect. 1.4 we recognize as a t-distribution with $(n-1)$ degrees of freedom. We therefore derive the correct $(1-\alpha)$-confidence interval

$$C = \left[\bar{X} - t_{1-\alpha/2}(n-1)\frac{S}{\sqrt{n}}, \ \bar{X} + t_{1-\alpha/2}(n-1)\frac{S}{\sqrt{n}}\right]$$

for the estimator $\bar{X}$ of the expected value. Again, this interval gets narrower if we increase the sample size n or decrease the variance σ^2 of the data.

As an example, let us repeatedly take 10 samples from a Norm(5,16) distribution and compute the corresponding 0.9-confidence interval for the estimated mean $\bar{X}$. For each such computation, we derive a slightly different interval, both in terms of the center of the interval (due to the estimated mean $\bar{X}$) and the length of the interval (due to the estimated variance of $\bar{X}$). For 25 repetitions, the confidence intervals are plotted next to each other in Fig. 2.2. Some intervals, such as the 5th and the 24th, do not cover the true value. To demonstrate the effect of estimating the variance, we compute the correct t-based and the incorrect normal confidence intervals, both using the estimated variance, for the 5th sample (which is too far away from the true mean) as

$$C^t = [1.396, 4.717] \quad \text{and} \quad C^{\text{norm}} = [0.631, 5.482].$$

The normal quantiles overestimate the width of the interval, such that the normal interval contains the true value, while the t-based does not.

2.3.1 The Bootstrap

For computing the confidence interval for a given estimate, we frequently encounter two problems: finding the variance of an estimator, and working out the distribution of an estimator that is not an MLE. In addition, the theory leading to normal (or t-based) confidence intervals is based on the asymptotic distribution of the estimator, which might be quite different than the distribution for small sample sizes. A very popular way for solving these problems is by using the *bootstrap* method, which aims at estimating all necessary quantities directly from the data themselves. While mainly used for computing the estimator's variance, the bootstrap method

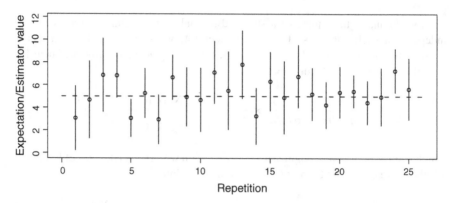

Fig. 2.2 Result of 25 repetitions of estimating the mean of a Norm(5,16) distribution, each with 10 samples. *Dashed line*: True value of mean $\mu = 5$, *solid lines*: 0.9-confidence intervals for estimators, points: estimated value of mean in ith repetition

also allows to compute higher moments, and even allows computation of confidence intervals for estimators with non-normal distribution.

Let us suppose we take b independent samples $Y_1, \ldots, Y_b$ from a distribution. Then, by the laws of large numbers, the sample mean approaches the true expectation for increasing b. The same argument still holds if we apply a function h on mean and expectation:

$$\frac{1}{b} \sum_{i=1}^{b} h(Y_i) \to \mathbb{E}(h(Y_1)).$$

For example, we recover the variance estimator by choosing $h = (Y_i - \bar{Y})^2$.

The key idea on how this helps is the following: let us consider any estimator $\hat{\theta}_n$ and denote by $F(x) = \mathbb{P}(\hat{\theta}_n \leq x)$ its cumulative distribution function. For the beginning, we are interested in calculating $\text{Var}(\hat{\theta}_n)$. This is comparatively easy if we know the distribution F of the estimator. If we do not, we can try to estimate this distribution by $\hat{F}$, and subsequently estimate the variance using this estimated distribution as an approximation. Let us assume we are given a set of data $x_1, \ldots, x_n$. For estimating $\hat{F}$, we re-sample new data from this given set, uniformly and with replacement, such that each x_i has the same probability to be re-sampled, and can also be re-sampled several times. We repeat this re-sampling b times, where $x_{j,1}^*, \ldots, x_{j,n}^*$ is the jth new sample. From each such sample, we compute the estimator $\hat{\theta}_{n,j}^*$, leading to a total of b estimates. Each sample is prone to be different from the others, and so are the estimated values.

If the data are a representative sample, this re-sampling gets us all the information needed: there are only few sample points with extreme values. These therefore get re-sampled rarely and are only present in a few bootstrap samples. On the other hand, "typical" values are sampled often, possibly even multiple times, into one bootstrap sample. The estimation is then performed more often on sets of "typical" data values than on more extreme, more unlikely combinations of values. This in turn gives a correct impression of how the estimator varies with varying data.

Overall, there are n^n different ways draw new samples of size n; this number is very large even for moderate n which ensures that we do get a different sample each time. The name "bootstrap" refers to the seemingly impossible task to lift ourselves out of the unknown variance problem by using the straps of our own boots, namely the data we have.

The algorithm. We can write the general bootstrap procedure for estimating the variance in a more algorithmic form as

- Draw $X_1^\star, \ldots, X_n^\star$ uniformly with replacement from $\{x_1, \ldots, x_n\}$.
- Compute $\hat\theta_{n,i}^\star = g(X_1^\star, \ldots, X_n^\star)$ from this bootstrap sample.
- Repeat the two steps b times to get the estimates $\hat\theta_{n,1}^\star, \ldots, \hat\theta_{n,b}^\star$.
- Compute the estimator's bootstrap variance estimate

$$\mathrm{Var}(\hat\theta_n) \approx v_{\mathrm{boot}} = \frac{1}{b} \sum_{i=1}^{b} \left(\hat\theta_{n,i}^\star - \frac{1}{b} \sum_{j=1}^{b} \hat\theta_{n,j}^\star \right)^2.$$

In R, the package boot offers a function boot() that simplifies the computation of statistics by the bootstrap method. Once the b bootstrapped values for $\hat\theta_n$ are computed, there are several ways to form a confidence interval.

The normal CI. If the estimator has a normal distribution, we may simply replace the variance $\mathrm{Var}(\hat\theta_n)$ by its bootstrap estimate v_{boot} and form the usual normal (or t-based) confidence interval

$$C^{\mathrm{norm}} = \hat\theta_n \pm z_{1-\alpha/2} \sqrt{v_{\mathrm{boot}}}.$$

The percentile CI. The second method relies on using the bootstrap samples of estimator values to compute the empirical quantile of its distribution and works for all unbiased estimators. For this, we sort the bootstrap estimates such that $\hat\theta_{n,(1)}^\star \leq \cdots \leq \hat\theta_{n,(b)}^\star$; again, the estimate with index (i) is the ith smallest one. Then for $k = b\alpha$ (suitably rounded to the next integer), $\hat\theta_\alpha^\star := \hat\theta_{n,(k)}^\star$ is the empirical α-quantile of the distribution of $\hat\theta_n$ and we form the empirical percentile confidence interval

$$C^{\mathrm{percentile}} = \left[\hat\theta_{\alpha/2}^\star, \hat\theta_{1-\alpha/2}^\star \right].$$

Example 16 Sometimes, the data are not normally distributed, but their logarithms are. The *log-normal distribution* with parameters μ and σ^2 is the distribution of $X = \exp(Y)$, with $Y \sim \mathrm{Norm}(\mu, \sigma^2)$. These parameters are the mean and variance of Y, but not of X. The distribution of X is asymmetric and we want to quantify this asymmetry using the skewness measure from Sect. 1.6.5. An unbiased estimator for the skewness θ of a sample is

Fig. 2.3 Density of
skewness estimates for
log-normal sample of size
500. Normal (*solid*) and pivot
(*dashed*) 0.95-confidence
intervals are given, computed
from $b = 100$ bootstrap
samples. The circle is the
original estimate of skewness

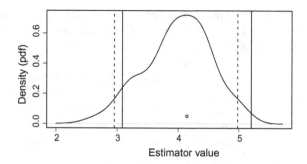

$$\hat{\theta}_n = \frac{\frac{1}{n}\sum_{i=1}^{n}(x_i - \bar{x})^3}{\left(\frac{1}{n}\sum_{i=1}^{n}(x_i - \bar{x})^2\right)^{\frac{3}{2}}}.$$

Instead of working out the distribution of this estimator, we apply the bootstrap method to derive the percentile and normal confidence interval for a given estimate.

For illustration, we generate $n = 500$ samples $X_1, \ldots, X_n$ of log-normal random variables with parameters $\mu = 0$, $\sigma = 1$. We then compute the skewness estimate $\hat{\theta}_n$, followed by $b = 100$ bootstrap samples from the X_i. Normal and pivot confidence intervals are finally computed for $\alpha = 0.05$.

The results are given in Fig. 2.3, where the estimate $\hat{\theta}_n$ is indicated by the small circle, and the normal and percentile 0.95-CIs are given by the solid and dashed lines, respectively. The solid black line gives the empirical density function of the estimator $\hat{\theta}_n$ estimated from the bootstrap samples. Interestingly, the percentile confidence interval is not symmetric around the estimate, because of a skewed estimator distribution.

2.4 Robust Estimation

There is one major problem with the estimators that we discussed so far: they all assume that each sample point is taken from the same underlying distribution, and there are thus no contaminations in the sample. A contamination can be an "outlier" that, by eye, can clearly be identified as an incorrect measurement, for example. Many estimators are very sensitive to such contaminations.

Example 17 A sample of $n = 20$ points from a Norm(5,4) is taken. In addition, the sample data is contaminated by only $n' = 2$ outliers, leading to the empirical density given in Fig. 2.4. Estimating the mean of the sample distribution gives the location indicated by the solid vertical line; it is substantially shifted to the right from the correct expected value which would be somewhere near the maximum of the density in this case.

To quantify how sensitive an estimator is to contaminations in the sample, the *robustness* of an estimator is measured by its *breakdown point*. It refers to the proportion of contaminations an estimator can handle before it gives arbitrarily large values. For the arithmetic mean, even one contamination has the capacity to make the estimate arbitrarily large, as even a single outlier very far away from the rest of the sample "pulls" the whole estimate away from the correct mean of the uncontaminated sample. Its breakdown point is therefore zero. The same argument holds for the two estimators for the variance, which both also have a breakdown point of zero.

While this might in practice not be as dramatic as theory suggests, simply because contaminations far away from the sample are often unlikely, it is nevertheless a reason to be uncomfortable, as it means that even a small amount of contamination can potentially yield very misleading results. For a small number of sample points, we might try a visual inspection to see if there are any unusual values in the sample, but this is clearly not a good strategy if we want to investigate large amounts of data. We will therefore investigate *robust estimators* with high breakdown points as alternatives for common estimators. Here, we will discuss robust alternatives for estimating the location and scale. They all rely on *order statistics* of the sorted sample, again denoted $x_{(1)} \leq \cdots \leq x_{(n)}$, and typically estimate empirical quantiles.

2.4.1 Location: Median and k-Trimmed Mean

Median. In addition to the expectation, the *median* is another measure for the location of a distribution. It corresponds to the 0.5-quantile $q_{0.5}$ of a distribution such that $\mathbb{P}(X \leq q_{0.5}) = 0.5$. We can estimate any α-quantile from the sorted sample simply by finding the correct index from $k = n\alpha$. If k is an integer, we simply select the kth smallest value, i.e., $\hat{q}(\alpha) = x_{(k)}$. If k is not an integer, we compute the two nearest integer k', k'' and interpolate the corresponding values $x_{(k')}$ and $x_{(k'')}$. Various ways for interpolation exist, many of which are implemented in the quantile() function in R. The estimate $\hat{q}(0.5)$ for the median is therefore simply the sample point in the middle (or the average of the two surrounding ones). As such, it does not use any information about the actual values of the sample points, but only uses information about the *rank*, i.e., their indices in the sorted sample.

Example 18 For $n = 8$ given sample points
$$6.39, 0.887, 1.521, 8.635, 7.742, 7.462, 6.631, 5.511,$$
the sorted values are
$$0.887, 1.521, 5.511, 6.39, 6.631, 7.462, 7.742, 8.635.$$

The median is estimated as $\hat{q}(0.5) = \frac{1}{2} \times (6.39 + 6.631) = 6.5105$ by interpolating between the two sample points with ranks 4 and 5.

Changing the largest value from 8.635 to 108.635 changes the mean substantially from $\hat{\mu} = 5.5974$ to $\hat{\mu}' = 18.0974$, but leaves the median unchanged at $\hat{q}'(0.5) = 6.5105$. In R, the median is computed by median().

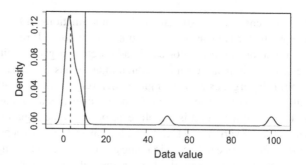

Fig. 2.4 Estimation of the location of a sample of 20 normally distributed points contaminated with 2 "outliers" with values 50 and 100. The true mean is $\mu = 5$. The two outliers "pull" the estimation of the mean to the right, leading to $\bar{x} = 10.72$ (*solid line*). The robust estimate of the median is $\hat{m}_{n+n'} = 3.82$ (*dashed line*), with a true median of 5

For the contaminated normal sample of Example 17, the estimated median $\hat{q}_{0.5} = 3.821$ is given by the dashed vertical line in Fig. 2.4. It is reasonably close to the true median $q_{0.5} = 5$ and largely unaffected by the two contaminations.

Let us look at the robustness of the median. We note that because it only considers ranks and not values, we can increase all points larger than the median arbitrarily without changing it. The same holds for decreasing smaller values and we conclude that the median has breakdown point 50%.

Both the mean and the median are measures for the location of the distribution, trying to give a single number to describe where "most" of the values are. The mean gives the expectation or average of a sample, wheres the median indicates the point such that half of the data is smaller (resp. larger). If the distribution is symmetric, the two values are identical, but they differ for skewed distributions. Because of its large breakdown point, the median is often the better choice for estimating the location. However, it cannot always be interpreted as the expected value of the distribution.

Trimmed means. If we still want to specifically estimate the expectation robustly, the k-trimmed mean is a good alternative to the median. It also uses the sorted values of the sample, but drops the k lowest and highest sample points of the data. The rationale is that contaminations are likely to be much smaller or much larger than the uncontaminated sample points. Formally,

$$\hat{\mu}(k) = \frac{1}{n - 2k} \sum_{i=k+1}^{n-k} x_{(i)}.$$

For $k = 0$, we recover the ordinary arithmetic mean again, for $k = n/2$ (taken to the next suitable integer), we recover the median. The k-trimmed mean is thus a generalization of both estimators. The choice for k is somewhat arbitrary of course, and should always be stated if this estimator is used; common choices are $k = 0.05 \times n$ and $k = 0.25 \times n$.

Example 19 For the 8 sample points of the previous example and $k = 1$, the k-trimmed mean reads

$$\hat{\mu}(1) = \frac{1}{8}(x_{(2)} + \cdots + x_{(7)}) = 5.876,$$

so the smallest and largest value are ignored and the ordinary arithmetic mean is computed from the remaining data. Again, changing the largest sample value from 8.635 to 108.635 does not change the estimate, as this point is ignored in the computation. In R, the k-trimmed mean can be accessed by mean(..., trim=...).

2.4.2 Scale: MAD and IQR

Similar considerations lead to two robust alternatives for measuring the scale of a distribution: the *median absolute deviation* (MAD) and the *inter-quartile-range* (IQR).

   Median absolute deviation. The MAD follows the same ideas as the variance, but measures the median of the absolute distance to the median:

$$MAD = median_i(|x_i - median_j(x_j)|).$$

   Inter-quartile range. The IQR computes the difference between the 0.25- and 0.75-quantile, and is given by the rectangle in a boxplot (see Sect. 1.8.4) that contains the medium 50% of the data:

$$IQR = q_{\frac{3}{4}} - q_{\frac{1}{4}}.$$

   Comparison to the variance. Both the MAD and the IQR give different measures for the scale compared to the variance. Similar to the median, they both are more based on the ranks and not the absolute values of the particular data, and have high breakdown points. For the normal distribution, $\sigma \approx 1.48 \times$ MAD, so variance and MAD are scaled versions of each other. In R, both MAD and IQR are easily accessible via the functions mad() and IQR().

Example 20 For $n = 20$ samples contaminated with $n' = 2$ "outliers" of Example 17, the various estimators are summarized in the following table. The second column gives the values estimated on the contaminated sample, the third column gives the values computed on the uncontaminated subset of the sample.

Estimator	Value	True value
$\bar{x} = \hat{\mu}$	11.19	4.81
$\hat{m} = q(0.5)$	4.39	4.28
$\hat{\mu}(\alpha = 0.1)$	5.11	4.62
$s = \hat{\sigma}$	22.12	1.95
IQR	2.46	1.52
MAD	1.23	1.07

As we would expect, the mean and the standard deviation give very different values on the contaminated and uncontaminated sample. In contrast, their robust counterparts all give estimates on the contaminated sample that are reasonably close to the uncontaminated values.

2.5 Minimax Estimation and Missing Observations

In addition to maximum-likelihood and least-squares, *minimax estimation* is a third principle to construct estimators.

2.5.1 Loss and Risk

Before introducing minimax estimation, let us briefly look into a theoretical frame-work that allows us to compare the performance of various estimators and derive new principles for their construction.

The *loss-function* $\mathcal{L}(\theta, \hat{\theta})$ measures the distance from the true parameter value and its estimate. Two popular choices for loss functions are the squared loss $\mathcal{L}(\theta, \hat{\theta}) = (\theta - \hat{\theta})^2$ and the absolute loss $\mathcal{L}(\theta, \hat{\theta}) = |\theta - \hat{\theta}|$.

The loss depends on the actual value of the estimator, and thus on the specific sample. To get a more general measure, we therefore look at the expected loss, known as the *risk* of the estimator

$$\mathcal{R}(\theta, \hat{\theta}) = \mathbb{E}(\mathcal{L}(\theta, \hat{\theta})).$$

For example, the risk of an unbiased estimator $\hat{\theta}$ with respect to the squared loss function is simply its variance:

$$\mathcal{R}(\theta, \hat{\theta}) = \mathbb{E}(\mathcal{L}(\theta, \hat{\theta})) = \mathbb{E}((\theta - \hat{\theta})^2) = \mathbb{E}((\hat{\theta} - \mathbb{E}(\hat{\theta}))^2).$$

A small risk indicates that on average, for all possible true parameter values, the estimator is not too far off.

Example 21   Let us calculate the risk for the maximum-likelihood estimator $\hat{p}_n$ of the matching probability p in the sequence matching example with respect to squared loss of the MLE $\hat{p}_n = M/n$:

$$\mathcal{R}(p, \hat{p}) = \mathbb{E}((\hat{p}_n - p)^2) = \text{Var}(\hat{p}_n) = \frac{p(1-p)}{n}.$$

As shown in Fig. 2.5 (solid line), the risk is highest for $p \approx 1/2$ and lowest for values near the boundary. Intuitively, for $p = 0$, we will not observe any matches, and always estimate correctly.

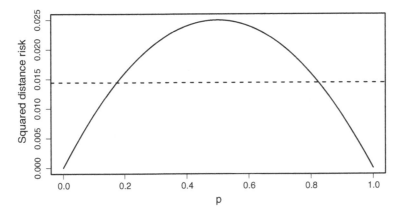

Fig. 2.5 Risk function for MLE $\hat{p}$ (*solid line*) and minimax estimator $\tilde{p}$ (*dashed line*) of the matching probability p

2.5.2 Minimax Estimators

For some applications, we might be interested in having a guarantee that the risk is not too high for any possible true value of the parameter. For this, we construct a *minimax estimator* $\tilde{\theta}$ such that the maximal risk

$$\max_{\theta} \; \mathscr{R}(\theta, \tilde{\theta})$$

is minimal. This means that while we allow the loss of this estimator to be larger for some values of θ, it will stay lower *on average* than any other estimator.

Example 22 Let us consider a different estimator for the matching example:

$$\tilde{p}_n = \frac{M + \frac{1}{2}\sqrt{n}}{n + \sqrt{n}}$$

has squared loss risk

$$\mathscr{R}(p, \tilde{p}_n) = \frac{n}{4(n + \sqrt{n})^2},$$

which is constant for all parameter values p and is smaller than the maximal risk of the MLE $\hat{p}_n$. Indeed, $\max_p \mathscr{R}(p, \hat{p}_n) = 1/4n$ but $\mathscr{R}(p, \tilde{p}_n) < 1/4n$ for all p, as one easily verifies. As we see in Fig. 2.5, however, the risk is not always lower than the MLE-risk, but is lower for mid-range parameter values and higher in the extremes.

Minimax estimators are also useful if some potential outcomes of an experiment have small probabilities and may not be observed due to a small sample size.

Example 23 Let us consider the following problem: the possible outcome of an experiment is one of s different types, such as A/C/G/T in the former random sequence examples, with each sequence position being one of the four possible nucleotides.

Such experiments are described by a *multinomial distribution*, which is a generalization of the binomial distribution to more than two outcomes. The probability for an observation of category i is p_i, and $\sum_{i=1}^{s} p_i = 1$. A result of such an experiment is a vector $(X_1, \ldots, X_s)$ containing the number of samples of category i in X_i, so that $\sum_{i=1}^{s} X_i = n$ is the total number of sample points.[1]

The probability mass function of $(X_1, \ldots, X_s)$ is given by

$$\mathbb{P}(X_1 = k_1, \ldots, X_s = k_s) = \frac{n!}{k_1! \cdots k_s!} p_1^{k_1} \cdots p_s^{k_s},$$

and the binomial distribution is recovered by setting $s = 2$, in which case $p_2 = 1 - p_1$ and $k_2 = n - k_1$, leading to the binomial coefficient. The expected number of observations in the ith category is $\mathbb{E}(X_i) = np_i$. In the sequence example, we would thus expect to see np_A A and np_G G in a sequence of length n. The probability of category i can be estimated by the maximum-likelihood estimator

$$\hat{p}_{n,i} = \frac{k_i}{n}.$$

A common rule-of-thumb suggests choosing a sample size n such that at least five observations are expected in each category for estimating the various probabilities with some confidence:

$$n \min_i(p_{n,i}) \geq 5 \Rightarrow n \geq \frac{5}{\min_i(p_{n,i})}.$$

For the possible nucleotides with probabilities

$$(p_A, p_C, p_G, p_T) = (1/2, 1/4, 1/8, 1/8),$$

we would thus need at least $5/0.125 = 40$ samples to reliably estimate all probabilities.

In practice, we usually do not know these probabilities, of course, and sometimes have no control over the possible sample size n. Imagine that we only have a sequence of 20 nucleotides. If it happens not to have any G, we consequently estimate $\hat{p}_G = 0$. This will have undesired consequences if we use these values for a model to describe the sequence matching probabilities, because the model would assume that G can never occur and will thus incorrectly predict the possible number of matchings.

One way of dealing with this problem is to introduce *pseudo-counts* by pretending that there is a certain number of observations in each category to begin with. For example, let us put a observations in each category before conducting the actual

---

[1]   Note that in contrast to the previous notation, all X_i together describe *one* experiment (or sample point).

experiment, and therefore see $x_i + a$ observations in category i after the experiment. Then, we can use the estimate

$$\tilde{p}_{n,i} = \frac{x_i + a}{sa + n}$$

for the categories' probabilities, which is simply the MLE for the modified data. With $a > 0$, each estimate is strictly larger than (but potentially very close to) zero.

Let us assume we observed $(x_A, x_C, x_G, x_T) = (13, 6, 0, 1)$. How large should we choose a? If we choose it too large, it would spoil the whole estimation and assign almost identical probabilities everywhere, independent of the data. For example, with $a = 1000$ the estimates are

$$(\tilde{p}_A, \tilde{p}_C, \tilde{p}_G, \tilde{p}_T) = (0.252, 0.25, 0.249, 0.249).$$

If we choose a too small, it might not have an effect and we end up with non-zero, but extremely low probabilities. Indeed, for $a = 0.1$,

$$(\tilde{p}_A, \tilde{p}_C, \tilde{p}_G, \tilde{p}_T) = (0.642, 0.299, 0.005, 0.054).$$

We can calculate a reasonable compromise by selecting a such that we minimize the maximal risk of the corresponding estimator. For parameters of the multinomial distribution, this minimax estimator is achieved by choosing

$$a = \frac{\sqrt{n}}{s}.$$

For the example, $a = 1.118$ and we estimate

$$(\tilde{p}_A, \tilde{p}_C, \tilde{p}_G, \tilde{p}_T) = (0.577, 0.291, 0.046, 0.087),$$

which is fairly close to the correct values, taking into account that we do not have many data available.

The seemingly ad-hoc estimator in Sect. 2.5.2 for the binomial case was derived in this way.

2.6 Fisher-Information and Cramér-Rao Bound

We conclude the chapter by a brief discussion of the idea of Fisher-information, from which we can derive a theoretical lower bound for the variance of an estimator. This bound tells us how precise we can actually estimate a given parameter with a fixed number of samples.

Recall the definition $\ell_n(\theta) = \sum_i \log(f(x_i; \theta))$ of the log-likelihood function. The *Fisher-score* is simply the derivative of this function with respect to the parameter(s),

$$\text{Fisher-score} = \frac{\partial \ell_n(\theta)}{\partial \theta},$$

and we calculate a maximum-likelihood estimator by finding its roots. In addition, the *Fisher-information* describes the curvature of the likelihood function around a parameter value θ. It is given by

$$I_n(\theta) = \sum_{i=1}^{n} \text{Var}\left(\frac{\partial \ell_n(\theta)}{\partial \theta}\right) = -n\mathbb{E}\left(\frac{\partial^2 \ell_n(\theta)}{\partial \theta^2}\right) = nI(\theta).$$

Loosely speaking, a large information indicates that the likelihood function will change noticeably when moving from θ to a nearby value θ'; the parameter value can then be estimated more reliably. A small information indicates a shallow "valley" in the likelihood function, where substantially different parameter values lead to almost identical values of $\ell_n(\theta)$.

Example 24 Let us again consider the matching example with log-likelihood function $\ell_n(p) = M \log(p) + (n - M) \log(1 - p)$ and

$$\frac{\partial \ell_n(p)}{\partial p} = \frac{M}{p} - \frac{n - M}{1 - p}.$$

The Fisher-information is

$$I_{n(p)} = -n\mathbb{E}\left(\frac{\partial^2 \ell_n(p)}{\partial p^2}\right) = -n\mathbb{E}\left(-\frac{M}{p^2} - \frac{n - M}{(1 - p)^2}\right)$$

$$= \frac{n}{p^2}\mathbb{E}(M) + \frac{n}{(1 - p)^2}\mathbb{E}(n - M) = \frac{n}{p(1 - p)}.$$

For sequences of length $n = 20$ nucleotides and $m = 12$ observed matches, the log-likelihood function and its Fisher-information are given in Fig. 2.6. As expected, the log-likelihood is highest at $p = m/n$. The Fisher-information does not take into consideration the actual observed matches and shows that for parameters p in the mid-range, the information carried by a sample is much lower than for more extreme parameter values near zero or one. This tells us that true values near the boundaries are much easier to estimate, as they lead to more dramatic expected changes in the likelihood function. These properties of the likelihood and information functions become more pronounced if we increase the number of samples from $n = 20$ to $n = 60$.

Cramér-Rao bound. The main importance of the Fisher-information is that it allows us to calculate the smallest possible variance that can be achieved with a given estimator and a given sample size. This *Cramér-Rao bound* states that

$$\text{Var}(\hat{\theta}_n) \geq \frac{1}{I_n(\theta)},$$

and we cannot decrease the variance of an estimator $\hat{\theta}_n$ below the reciprocal of its information. For getting estimates with lower variance and thus, for example,

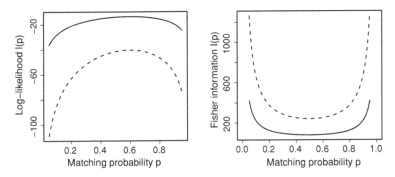

Fig. 2.6 Log-likelihood function $\ell_n(p)$ (*left*) and Fisher information $I_n(p)$ (*right*) for the sequence matching example with $n = 20$ and $m = 12$ observed matches (*solid lines*) and $n = 60, m = 36$ (*dashed lines*)

narrower confidence intervals, we either need to increase the sample size (because $I_n(\theta) \approx nI(\theta)$) or choose another estimator. Indeed, some estimators can be shown to have lowest variance among all other estimators for the same parameters.

2.7 Summary

Estimation allows us to infer the value of various properties of a distribution, such as its location, from data. We can construct corresponding estimators by the maximum-likelihood, the least-squares, and the minimax approach. Estimators are random variables because their realization depends on a given random sample. Their properties such as consistency and unbiasedness allow us to compare different estimators.

For a concrete estimation, we can compute confidence intervals around the estimated value to quantify how good the estimate is. These intervals contain the true value with high probability. For their computation, we need to know the distribution of the estimator to find the corresponding quantiles, and its standard error to scale correctly. The bootstrap offers a practical method to establish confidence intervals by resampling the data and computing empirical quantiles from the corresponding estimated values.

The breakdown point describes the sensitivity of an estimator to contaminations in the data. Because many classical estimators have a very low breakdown point, we should usually try to use robust alternatives, such as the median. Many robust estimators are based on the ranks of sample points rather than their values.

Missing observations and small sample sizes can cause major problems when estimating multinomial probabilities. Using minimax estimation to calculate pseudo-counts enables us to partly circumvent these problems.

Chapter 3
Hypothesis Testing

Abstract Testing provides the formal framework to reject or not reject a hypothesis on parameters, depending on whether it is supported by given data. Test levels and p-values allow to quantify the chances of false rejections due to the randomness of the data. Correct interpretation of test results is discussed in more detail and methods to adjust the probability of false rejections for multiple testing are presented.

Keywords Hypotheses · p-value · Multiple testing · FDR

> *Are the effects of A and B different? They are always*
> *different—for some decimal place*
>
> John Tukey

3.1 Introduction

A typical testing problem is the following: to decide if and which new treatment works better than a standard treatment, a group of patients is given the new treatment, while a *control group* is given the standard treatment. The time until recovery is recorded for each patient and a new treatment is considered better if the average recovery time is considerably shorter than that of the control group. The problem is to quantify what we mean by "considerably shorter", as the average times are computed from a random sample and although the new treatment might be better, the controls patient might— just by chance—nevertheless recover in comparable time: by visual inspection of the results shown in Fig. 3.1, it seems that treatments A and B work better than the control, but just by visual inspection, no clear decision can be made.

In this chapter, we investigate *statistical hypothesis testing* to formally describe the hypothesis to be tested (e.g., new treatment works better) and compare it with an alternative (e.g., new treatment works not better). Hypothesis testing will allow us to capture that one of the hypotheses is correct but just by chance, the data suggests otherwise. Quantifying these probabilities leads to the concept of *statistical significance*.

H.-M. Kaltenbach, *A Concise Guide to Statistics*, SpringerBriefs in Statistics,   53
DOI: 10.1007/978-3-642-23502-3_3, © Hans-Michael Kaltenbach 2012

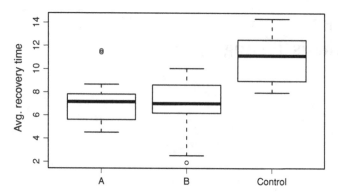

Fig. 3.1 Recovery times of patients for three different treatments Control, A, B. While both treatments A and B seems to be superior to the control, a potential difference between A and B is much less pronounced

Example 25 Let us first come back to the sequence matching example, where $M \sim \text{Binom}(n, p_0)$ is the number of matches of two random, unrelated sequences of fixed length n, and $p_0 = p_A^2 + p_C^2 + p_G^2 + p_T^2$ is the probability of seeing a match in any given position.

Assume we observe m matches in a pair of such sequences and want to conclude whether or not these sequences are related. In Example 8, we argued that if m is substantially larger than $\mathbb{E}(M)$ for unrelated sequences (thus using p_0 as matching probability), we have good reason to claim that the sequences are related and the number of matches then follows a $\text{Binom}(n, p)$ distribution with a higher matching probability $p > p_0$, leading also to a higher expected number of matches. Another way of deciding whether the sequences are related is therefore to ask whether the true matching probability p and the theoretical probability p_0 for the case of unrelated sequences are different. Of course, we do not know the correct probability p, so we have to work with its estimate $\hat{p}_n$. To test our hypothesis, we therefore need to decide whether the observed matching probability deviates substantially from the predicted probability p_0. Because $\hat{p}_n = M/n$ is a random variable, we can use its distribution to figure out how likely it is to observe a certain estimate $\hat{p}_n = m/n$ under the assumption that the true parameter value is p_0.

For simplicity, let us assume that $p_A = p_C = p_G = p_T = 1/4$ and consequently $p_0 = 1/4$ for unrelated sequences. Let us further denote by H_0 the hypothesis that the sequences are unrelated, so the true parameter p is the same as in the model for unrelated sequences:

$$H_0 : p = p_0 = \frac{1}{4}.$$

We would like to calculate whether the observed data give evidence *against* this *null hypothesis* and *in favor* of an *alternative hypothesis* H_1. Several alternative hypotheses are possible, for example

- the *simple* alternative $H_1 : p = 0.35$,
- the *composite* and *one-sided* alternative $H_1 : p > \frac{1}{4}$,
- the *composite* and *two-sided* alternative $H_1 : p \neq \frac{1}{4}$.

Each of these alternatives claims that the probability for a match in the two sequences is a certain parameter p, and gives valid ranges for this parameter. While the simple alternative claims a specific value, the composite alternatives give whole ranges of feasible values. More general, we can also define two (disjoint) sets Θ_0 and Θ_1 such that the null- and alternative hypotheses are $H_0 : p \in \Theta_0$ and $H_1 : p \in \Theta_1$, respectively.

Intuitively, consider sequences of length $n = 1000$ with $m = 100$ observed matches. With $\hat{p}_n = 1/10$, this indicates that the matching probability is actually much smaller than $p_0 = 1/4$. However, with the alternative $H_1 : p > 1/4$, this data would not give evidence against H_0. This does not mean that H_0 is true (which clearly isn't the case here), but that the alternative H_1 cannot explain the data any better than H_0. On the contrary, if we test H_0 against the two-sided alternative $H_1 : p \neq 1/4$, there is sufficient evidence that this alternative provides a better explanation for the data, so we would reject the null hypothesis.

To make these considerations more quantitative and rigorous, let us use the one-sided alternative $H_1 : p > 1/4$, so we only need to check if we observe unusually many (and not perhaps unusually few) matches. Consider the following argument: if H_1 is true, we expect to see more matches than if H_0 were true. However, the number of matches is random, and there is the possibility that even if H_0 is true, the observed counts are high just by chance. Knowing the distribution of M under H_0 (i.e., with $p = p_0 = 1/4$), we can compute the probability that M exceeds an observed number m of matches under H_0; this is the probability that the distribution stated in H_0 gives rise to data at least as extreme as observed. If this probability is very low, this indicates that the null hypothesis is unlikely to be true, as it is unlikely that the data have been generated with the stated parameters.

We know that the number of matches has a Binomial distribution. If the null hypothesis is true, we also know that the matching parameter p is equal to $p_0 = 1/4$. With this information, we compute the probability to see at least the observed number of m matches, provided the null hypothesis is indeed correct, to be

$$\mathbb{P}(M \geq m | H_0) = 1 - \mathbb{P}(M < m | H_0) = 1 - \sum_{i=0}^{m-1} \binom{n}{i} p_0^i (1 - p_0)^{n-i},$$

where we slightly abuse the notation for conditional probabilities for brevity.

For Example 8, we considered sequences of length $n = 100$ and $m = 29$ observed matches. The probability to see at least this number of matches in unrelated sequences is $\mathbb{P}(M \geq 29 | H_0) = 0.1495$, which gives no evidence against H_0 in favor of H_1. On the contrary, the probability to observe at least $m = 50$ matches in unrelated sequences is $\mathbb{P}(M \geq 50 | H_0) = 2.13e - 08$, providing substantial evidence that H_0 is actually false.

The calculated probabilities $\mathbb{P}(M \geq m | H_0)$ are called *p-values*. To reject or not reject a given null hypothesis, we fix a probability α and compute a threshold c such that $\mathbb{P}(M \geq c | H_0) = \alpha$. We then *reject* H_0 in favor of H_1, if $m > c$ and *do not reject* if $m \leq c$, leading to the *rejection region* $\mathcal{R}_\alpha = (c, \infty)$. The probability α describes the *false positive* errors, as it is the probability that we reject H_0, although it is actually correct. For the example with sequence length $n = 100$ and a probability of $\alpha = 0.05$, we calculate

$$\mathbb{P}(M \geq c | H_0) = \begin{cases} 0.0693, & \text{for } c = 32, \\ 0.0446, & \text{for } c = 33. \end{cases}$$

We would therefore use the more conservative $c = 33$ as our threshold, reject H_0 : $p = 1/4$ in favor of $H_1 : p > 1/4$ in the case $m = 50 > c$, and not reject in the case $m = 29 < c$.

Importantly, not rejecting is not the same as *accepting* H_0 because if we do not have evidence against H_0, we cannot conclude that it is actually true. We should therefore never speak of "accepting" the null hypothesis, but only of "not rejecting".

3.2 The General Procedure

The considerations taken in the introductory example can be divided in the following steps, providing the general setup for testing statistical hypotheses.

1. Clarify assumptions on independence, sample sizes etc. This will guide the choices in the next steps and is usually only done implicitly.
2. Formulate the *null hypothesis* H_0 and the *alternative hypothesis* H_1.
   Choose H_0 such that we retain it unless there is strong evidence against it. Choose H_1 to be simple or composite and one- or two-sided depending on the problem.
3. Choose a *test statistic* $T = g(X_1, \ldots, X_n)$ as a function of the data X_i.
4. Derive the *null-distribution* of T, i.e., its distribution $\mathbb{P}(T \leq t | H_0)$ under the assumption that H_0 holds.
   This is usually the difficult part. Of course, the choice of T above is already partially guided by the necessity to determine its null-distribution. For many practical purposes, steps 3 and 4 are done simply by looking up the appropriate test.
5. Compute the test statistic's value $t = g(x_1, \ldots, x_n)$ from the data $x_1, \ldots, x_n$.
6. Compute the *p-value* $\mathbb{P}(T \geq t | H_0)$.
   The smaller the *p*-value, the less likely it is that the observed value t was generated from the null-distribution.

Ultimately, the *p*-value gives us the information to either reject or don't reject the null hypothesis in favor of the alternative hypothesis. To arrive at such a decision from a given *p*-value, we decide on a *level* α for the test. This level gives the probability of getting a false positive, i.e., of falsely rejecting H_0 although it is true, due to uncommonly large deviations of the observed test statistic t from the expected value under H_0. Using this level, we then compute the rejection region $\mathcal{R}_\alpha$ of T such that we reject the null hypothesis if the observed value t is inside the *rejection region* $\mathcal{R}_\alpha$, and do not reject if it is outside. This rejection region is computed from the distribution of T under H_0 and the two hypotheses. If the null hypothesis is rejected at a level α, we say that the test is *significant at level α*.

The p-value corresponds to the smallest level α such that the test would not yet reject. For example, if we observe a p-value of 0.034, the test would reject at the $\alpha = 0.05$ level, but not at the $\alpha = 0.01$ level. Indeed, no R-implementation of a statistical test requires a test level; they all report the p-value, so we can decide what to do.

Absence of evidence is not evidence of absence. Rejecting the null hypothesis hinges on the distribution of the test statistic *assuming H_0 is true*. The p-value gives the probability that we see a value at least as extreme as the observed one under this distribution. It is *not* the probability that H_0 is true. A very low p-value indicates that the test statistic is unlikely to take the observed value under H_0 and therefore provides good reason to reject it. On the contrary, a high p-value does not give proof that H_0 is actually true. In fact, it could be that the alternative just provides an even worse explanation, or the test has very low power to distinguish the two alternatives.

As a consequence, a statistical test should always be stated such that the null hypothesis defines the "status quo" and gets rejected if the desired result shows in the data. Thus, testing for a difference between a default and non-default assumption, we would set H_0 to state that there is no difference and reject this hypothesis in favor of the alternative that there is a difference. This way, we can quantify our level of confidence in the rejection by a low p-value. Would we set the no difference scenario as alternative, we would aim at "proving" H_0 with the data, which we can't.

Very informally, let T be our test statistic with value t for some specific data. Then, we compute $\mathbb{P}(T \geq t | H_0)$, the probability to see this data if H_0 is true, which is not $\mathbb{P}(H_0 | T \geq t)$, the probability of H_0 being true, given the data.

Stating the hypotheses. Stating a null hypothesis H_0 to reflect the default assumptions can become quite intricate for more involved problems. In particular, it might not be straightforward to formulate the hypothesis in terms of parameter regions or even to find the formal statistical hypothesis that correctly reflects our verbal hypothesis on the data. This lead some researchers to introduce a *type-III error* (see Sect. 3.5 for type-I/II errors), which is often stated as "asking the wrong question and using the wrong H_0", or "correctly rejecting H_0, but for the wrong reasons".

Additionally, we have also to take some care in stating a useful alternative hypothesis. As we already saw, the choice of the alternative partly determines the rejection region. For the case of one mean μ, the decision for a two- or a one-sided alternative can usually be decided from the problem itself. However, imagine we were to test two means at the same time with null hypothesis $H_0 : \mu_A > 0, \mu_B > 0$. A reasonable alternative is $H_1 : \mu_A < 0, \mu_B < 0$, but it is very strict and we may want to relax it to $H_1 : (\mu_A < 0 \text{ or } \mu_B < 0)$. Depending on which alternative we select, this leads to different rejection regions.

3.3 Testing the Mean of Normally Distributed Data

One of the most frequent applications of statistical testing involves questions about the location of a distribution. In particular, we are often interested whether the mean of a given sample deviates significantly from an assumed value or whether two samples have the same mean. A typical example is the comparison of the result of an experiment to a control. This control can either be an assumed model, predicting the mean, or another experiment. In this section, we will discuss statistical tests to answer these questions with decreasing amount of additional assumptions. We start with a pedagogical example where we assume the distribution to be normal and the variance to be known, before introducing the family of t-tests which allow us to use estimates for the variance.

These tests are not applicable for non-normal data and we should always check the data for normality before performing any of them. We can do this visually using a normal quantile-quantile plot as introduced in Sect. 1.8.3. If the empirical quantiles do not deviate too much from the straight line expected from a normal distribution, it is usually safe to use a t-test. Of course, "too much" deviation is pretty subjective and one should always provide the Q-Q-plot in addition to the test results. For a more quantitative check, we might use the Kolmogorov-Smirnov test for testing normality in the data (Sect. 3.4.1) or the more specialized Shapiro-Wilks test (Sect. 3.4.2).

While not directly testing the mean, the *Wilcoxon-test* is often used for similar purposes on non-normally distributed data; it will be introduced in Sect. 3.4.3. We also only consider the two-sample case with independent data. If the two samples happen to be paired, for example, by measuring the weight of the same set of people before and after a treatment and comparing the two values for each patient, a *paired t-test* needs to be used.

3.3.1 Known Variance

Let us assume that we measure the weights $x_1, \ldots, x_n$ of n people from a particular region. We claim that people are substantially heavier in this region than a particular weight μ_0. Thus, our two hypotheses are informally "H_0 : weights are pretty much μ_0" versus "H_1 : weights are larger than μ_0". Note that the case of weights lower than μ_0 is not covered.

Clarifying assumptions. We assume that we have reason to believe (or actually checked) that the measured weights follow a normal distribution, so $X_i \sim \text{Norm}(\mu, \sigma^2)$. For simplicity, we further assume that we know the variance σ^2 and do not need to estimate it from the data. Clearly, this is often an unrealistic assumption, and we will discard it in Sect. 3.3.2.

Formulating the hypotheses. The two hypotheses can be formally written as

$$H_0 : \mu = \mu_0$$
$$H_1 : \mu > \mu_0,$$

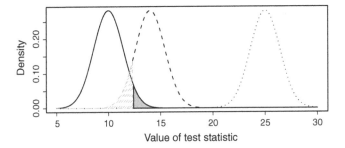

Fig. 3.2 Distribution of test statistic $\bar{X}$ under $H_0 : \mu = \mu_0 = 10$ (*solid*) and two values for the alternative: $\mu = 14$ (*dashed*) and $\mu = 25$ (*dotted*). Shaded areas correspond to a false positive probability of $\alpha = 0.05$ (*solid gray*) and to a false negative probability of 0.118 for a true value $\mu = 14$ (*dashed gray*)

or equivalently

$$H_0 : \mu - \mu_0 = 0$$
$$H_1 : \mu - \mu_0 > 0.$$

The alternative is composite, as it encompasses a set of possible values, and one-sided, as it ignores the possibility that the data is actually smaller than the claimed value.

Choosing the test statistic. Since we do not know the true mean μ, we estimate it by $\bar{x} = \hat{\mu}_n$, and thus compare a random number with the claimed mean μ_0. This is an example where we use an estimator as the test statistic.

Deriving the distribution under H_0. As an MLE, the arithmetic mean $\bar{X}$ itself has a normal distribution with parameters $\mathbb{E}(\bar{X}) = \mu$ and $\text{Var}(\bar{X}) = \sigma^2/n$ (this is where the known variance comes into play: the normal distribution is only correct if we do not need to estimate the variance).

Fixing a test level α, and thus the allowed probability for a false positive, only requires the distribution of $\bar{X}$ under H_0, which in this case is $\bar{X} \sim \text{Norm}(\mu_0, \sigma^2/n)$. The composite alternative describes a whole family of distributions, namely all normal distributions with variance σ^2/n and any mean $\mu > \mu_0$.

In Fig. 3.2, the distributions of $\bar{X}$ for $n = 20$ sample points and a variance of $\sigma^2 = 40$ are shown for a true mean of $\mu = 10$ (solid line), of $\mu = 14$ (dashed line), and of $\mu = 25$ (dotted line). Testing $\mu = \mu_0 = 10$ thus leads to the null distribution depicted by a solid line, while the dashed and dotted lines describe two distributions out of infinitely many given in the alternative hypothesis.

Computing the rejection region. For an observed arithmetic mean $\bar{x}$, the p-value for the test is $\mathbb{P}(\hat{\mu}_n \geq \bar{x}|H_0) = 1 - \Phi(\bar{x}; \mu_0, \sigma^2/n)$. Let us fix a test level of $\alpha = 0.05$. The rejection region is easily calculated as (c, ∞), where c is the value such that $\mathbb{P}(\bar{X} \geq c|H_0) = 0.05$, which computes to

$$c = \mu_0 + z_{1-\alpha}\frac{\sigma}{\sqrt{n}}.$$

For the proposed α, we have $z_{0.95} = 1.645$, which for $\mu_0 = 10$ leads to the rejection region

$$\mathscr{R}_{0.95} = (12.326, \infty),$$

and we reject $H_0 : \mu = \mu_0 = 10$ if $\bar{x} > 12.326$. For smaller differences, we do not reject.

The probability of a false positive for the level $\alpha = 0.05$ is given in Fig. 3.2 by the solid gray area. For a true value of $\mu = 14$, this level leads to probability of 0.118 for a false negative (H_0 not rejected although false), given by the dashed gray area, and a false positive probability of 0 for a true value of $\mu = 25$. We will come back to these two error probabilities in Sect. 3.5.

Equivalently, we can conclude that the normalized difference of observed and claimed mean has a standard normal distribution,

$$T := \frac{\bar{X} - \mu_0}{\sqrt{\frac{1}{n}}\sigma} \sim \text{Norm}(0, 1), \tag{3.1}$$

and we reject if its realization t exceeds the corresponding quantile, i.e., if

$$t > z_{1-\alpha}.$$

The two-sided alternative. If we test against the two-sided alternative $H_1 : \mu \neq \mu_0$, the rejection region consists of two intervals, which contain values that are considered too low and too high, respectively. Very similar to before, the rejection region $\mathscr{R}_\alpha = (-\infty, c_1) \cup (c_2, +\infty)$ is computed such that

$$\mathbb{P}(\bar{X} \in \mathscr{R}_\alpha | H_0) = \alpha$$

holds, which immediately leads to

$$\mathscr{R}_\alpha = \left(-\infty, \mu_0 + z_{\alpha/2}\frac{\sigma}{\sqrt{n}}\right) \cup \left(\mu_0 + z_{1-\alpha/2}\frac{\sigma}{\sqrt{n}}, +\infty\right).$$

We thus reject H_0 if $\bar{x} \in \mathscr{R}_\alpha$, or, equivalently, if $|T| > z_{1-\alpha/2}$, with T the normalized difference defined by (3.1). For the level $\alpha = 0.05$ and parameters as before, the two critical thresholds are $c_1 = 7.228$ and $c_2 = 12.772$.

Rejection regions and confidence intervals. There is a striking similarity between the rejection region $\mathscr{R}_\alpha$ of the test statistic T and the $(1 - \alpha)$-confidence interval of the estimator $\bar{X}$ for the mean. Indeed, if we use any estimator $\hat{\theta}_n$ directly as the test statistic, we reject the null hypothesis $H_0 : \theta = \theta_0$ at the level α if θ is not contained in the $(1 - \alpha)$-confidence interval of $\hat{\theta}_n$.

3.3.2 Unknown Variance: t-Tests

Clearly, the assumption that we do not know the mean of a sample—but exactly know the variance—is an oversimplification in most practical cases. We will therefore drop this assumption and additionally estimate the variance from the data, which leads to the t-distribution under the null hypothesis. The corresponding family of tests is then known as t-test. We describe these tests for three cases: (i) we test one sample mean for a specific value, but need to estimate the variance, (ii) we test if the means of two samples are equal, with both samples having the same, but unknown variance, (iii) we test if the means of two samples are equal, each sample having unknown variance.

We will again assume that the data $X_1, \ldots, X_n$ (and $Y_1, \ldots, Y_m$ for the two-sample cases) are normally distributed with means μ_X and μ_Y, and variances σ_X^2 and σ_Y^2, respectively.

One sample with unknown variance. Let us consider n sample points from a Norm(μ_X, σ_X^2) distribution, where both the mean μ_X and the variance σ_X^2 are unknown and need to be estimated. We estimate σ_X^2 as before by

$$S_X^2 = \hat{\sigma}_X^2 = \frac{1}{n-1} \sum_{i=1}^{n} (X_i - \bar{X})^2.$$

To test the hypothesis $H_0 : \mu_X = \mu_0$, we can again use the normalized difference

$$T = \frac{\bar{X} - \mu_0}{\sqrt{\frac{1}{n} S_X}}$$

between observed and expected mean as test statistic, this time replacing the variance by its estimate. The test statistic T does *not* have a normal distribution, but a t-distribution with $n - 1$ degrees of freedom. The reason for this is exactly the same as for computing the confidence interval for the mean's estimator $\bar{X}$ with estimated variance: the estimate of the mean from the data became more uncertain, leading to slightly heavier tails of the distribution. We consequently reject in favor of the two-sided alternative $H_1 : \mu_X \neq \mu_0$ if the normalized difference of claimed and observed mean is too large and the absolute value of the test statistic therefore exceeds the corresponding t-quantile:

$$\text{Reject } H_0 \iff |T| > t_{1-\alpha/2}(n - 1),$$

and similarly for the one-sided alternatives.

Example 26 With 10 random samples from a Norm(15, 40) distribution, the test $H_0 : \mu_X = 10$ against the two-sided alternative $H_1 : \mu_X \neq 10$ gives a p-value of 0.02262 for the t-test, but a too low p-value of 0.00302 when using the normal distribution with estimated variance.

Two samples with unknown and unequal variances. In practice, one is often interested in testing whether two samples differ significantly in their mean rather than testing one sample mean against a given value. As an example, we might have some data X_i from an experiment and some data Y_i from a control, and ask whether there is any difference in the samples' means. This is known as a *two-sample* test problem. Formally, we like to test $H_0 : \mu_X = \mu_Y$ against the alternative, e.g., $H_1 : \mu_X \neq \mu_Y$. Moreover, the samples are allowed to be of different size. As before, our test statistic will be the difference of the two estimated means. Because both estimators are maximum-likelihood and therefore have a normal distribution, their difference is also normally distributed. The only thing we need to figure out is the variance of this difference, so we can normalize correctly to get a standard normal distribution for the estimator. Recalling the elementary properties of the variance, the variance of the difference is quickly established:

$$\mathrm{Var}(\bar{X} - \bar{Y}) = \mathrm{Var}(\bar{X}) + \mathrm{Var}(-\bar{Y}) + 2\mathrm{Cov}(\bar{X}, \bar{Y}) = \mathrm{Var}(\bar{X}) + \mathrm{Var}(\bar{Y}),$$

because the X and Y samples are independent and thus $\mathrm{Cov}(\bar{X}, \bar{Y}) = 0$. Thus,

$$\widehat{\mathrm{Var}}(\bar{X} - \bar{Y}) = \frac{S_X^2}{n} + \frac{S_Y^2}{m}$$

is an estimator for the variance of the difference, which immediately leads to the test statistic

$$T = \frac{\bar{X} - \bar{Y}}{\sqrt{\frac{1}{n}S_X^2 + \frac{1}{m}S_Y^2}}.$$

However, computing the correct distribution of this test statistic is quite tedious and yields a formula that contains the true parameter values, which are of course not available. In practice, this distribution is therefore approximated by a *t*-distribution with ν (or less) degrees of freedom, where ν is computed as

$$\nu = \frac{\left(\frac{S_X^2}{n} + \frac{S_Y^2}{m}\right)^2}{\frac{S_X^4}{\frac{n^2}{n-1}} + \frac{S_Y^4}{\frac{m^2}{m-1}}},$$

and we reject $H_0 : \mu_X = \mu_Y$ if $|T| > t_{1-\alpha/2}(\nu)$ in favor of $H_1 : \mu_X \neq \mu_Y$. Most implemented versions of this test, such as the function t.test() in R, automatically decide on the correct test statistic and the relevant parameters.

Two samples with unknown but equal variances. If the two variances are expected to be equal or at least very similar, we can replace the two individual estimates S_X^2 and S_Y^2 by the *pooled variance*

$$S_{XY}^2 = \frac{(n-1)S_X^2 + (m-1)S_Y^2}{n+m-2}.$$

This estimate looks quite similar to the usual estimate of a variance: we "lost" two degrees of freedom, one for each arithmetic mean and consequently divide by the total degrees of freedom from the overall sample, $m+n-2$. The test statistic is again the difference of the two observed means, normalized by the standard deviation of this difference:

$$T = \frac{\bar{X} - \bar{Y}}{\sqrt{\frac{1}{n} + \frac{1}{m}} S_{XY}}.$$

This test statistic has a t-distribution with $m + n - 2$ degrees of freedom and we reject $H_0 : \mu_X = \mu_Y$ if $|T| > t_{1-\alpha/2}(m + n - 2)$ in favor of $H_1 : \mu_X \neq \mu_Y$.

Example 27 As a very brief example, let us look at a t-test performed on two sets of samples with $n = 10$ samples from a Norm(10, 40) distribution and $m = 13$ samples from a Norm(12, 30) distribution. In practice, we would not know the correct distributions and want to test whether the two sample means differ significantly. For this, we perform a two-sided t-test with null hypothesis $H_0 : \mu_X - \mu_Y = 0$ versus the alternative $H_1 : \mu_X - \mu_Y \neq 0$. Using the R implementation of this test, we get the following report:

```
          Welch Two Sample t-test

data: x and y
t = -2.0876, df = 15.988, p-value = 0.0532
alternative hypothesis: true difference in means is not
equal to 0
95 percent confidence interval:
 -9.96370876 0.07680932
sample estimates:
mean of x mean of y
 7.705368 12.648818
```

In the first line, R informs us that it uses a variant of the t-test, known as the Welch-test, here in its two-sample form. It then reports the data used, the values for the test statistic, the estimated degrees of freedom, and the p-value. We note that the degrees of freedom are not integer, but were calculated using an interpolation formula due to the different sample sizes and variances. After giving the alternative used, it reports the 95% confidence interval for the test statistic and finally the two estimated means. Note that the confidence interval is for the difference in means and should contain 0, if the means are the same. The test gives a p-value of 0.0532, which is significant at the $\alpha = 0.1$, but not the $\alpha = 0.05$ level.

3.4 Other Tests

Apart from testing the mean of one or two samples, there are many more hypotheses that can be tested using suitable test statistics. In this section, we will introduce a small variety of such tests and briefly explain their major ideas.

3.4.1 Testing Equality of Distributions: Kolmogorov-Smirnov

The *Kolmogorov-Smirnov (KS) test* checks whether a sample follows a given distribution (one-sample version) or if two samples are equally distributed (two-sample version). The test statistic is the maximal difference (technically: the supremum of the difference) of the empirical cumulative distribution function and the given distribution function:

$$D := \sup_x \left| \hat{F}_n(x) - F(x) \right|.$$

This difference takes values between zero and one and is larger, the more the sample distribution deviates from the given one.

The KS-test works for any distribution. However, the distribution function F has to be completely specified by explicitly stating all parameter values.

The two-sample version tests the two empirical cdfs $\hat{F}$ and $\hat{G}$:

$$D := \sup_x \left| \hat{F}_n(x) - \hat{G}_n(x) \right|.$$

An example is given in Fig. 3.3, where 20 exponentially distributed sample points are generated for $\lambda = 3$ and their ecdf compared to the cdf of a normal distribution with parameters $\mu = 0.5$ and $\sigma^2 = 0.1$. The largest difference is $D = 0.3983$ found at $x = 0.4213$, leading to a p-value of $p = 0.002248$. This indicates strong evidence against the null hypothesis and we would conclude that the distributions are indeed different.

3.4.2 Testing for Normality: Shapiro-Wilks

Normality of the data is a very common assumption for statistical tests and procedures. The *Shapiro-Wilks test* provides a more specialized alternative to the Kolmogorov-Smirnov test for testing if the data is indeed normally distributed. This test compares the variance of the data, estimated as $s^2 = 1/(n-1) \sum_i (x_i - \bar{x})^2$, with the variance expected by a normal distribution. For computing this expected variance b^2, the test uses the same method as a normal Q-Q-plot and estimates the

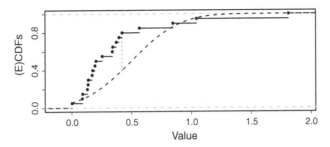

Fig. 3.3 Kolmogorov-Smirnov test. The empirical cdf of 20 Exp(3) samples (*black dots and lines*) is compared to the theoretical Norm(0.5, 0.1) cdf (*dashed line*). The test statistic measures the largest absolute difference $D = 0.3983$, found here at 0.4213 and denoted by a *dotted vertical line*

slope of the normal Q-Q-line (see Sect. 1.8.3). The test statistic is then the quotient of the two variances

$$W = \frac{b^2}{(n-1)s^2},$$

and we test $H_0 : W = 1$, expected if the data is normal, against $H_1 : W \neq 1$. This test generally performs better than the corresponding KS-test and should be preferred, especially for small sample sizes. A sample size of $n \geq 3$ is necessary for the test to work, and an upper limit is given with $n \approx 3000$.

3.4.3 Testing Location: Wilcoxon

For testing whether two distributions are equal, we can also rely on another non-parametric test known as the *Wilcoxon* or *Mann-Whitney-U* test. While not testing the location itself but rather the whole distributions, this test can nevertheless often be used as a non-parametric alternative to the *t*-test family if the data is not normally distributed, provided the variances in the samples are of comparable size and the sample distributions are similar enough such that the differences are mainly caused by different locations.

The main idea of the Wilcoxon test is the following: let us again assume that $X_1, \ldots, X_n$ and $Y_1, \ldots, Y_m$ are two samples of size n and m, respectively, and let us again denote by $X_{(i)}$ the ith smallest sample point, which we say to have rank i. We now join the samples into a new sample Z and denote by $Z_{(i)}$ the ith smallest sample point in the joint sample, so i runs from 1 to $n + m$. Provided the two samples have similar distributions, the ranks of the two individual samples within the joint sample should distribute equally and we expect to see a good "mixing" of the two samples in Z.

The Wilcoxon test now compares the sum of the ranks of X and Y in Z to decide whether this is indeed the case. For this, let us denote by R_X the sum of all ranks of elements of the X sample in the ordered joint sample Z. In practice, we check whether $Z_{(i)}$ originally belonged to the X and if so, we add i to the sum, until we reach the $(m + n)$th element of Z. Similary, let us denote by R_Y the sum of ranks of the Y samples in Z, established by the same procedure.

The sum of all ranks is then

$$R_X + R_Y = \sum_{i=1}^{n+m} i = \frac{(n + m)(n + m + 1)}{2},$$

and the first sample of size n provides the fraction $\frac{n}{n+m}$ of the joint sample. Further, R_X is bounded by

$$\sum_{i=1}^{n} i = \frac{n(n + 1)}{2} \leq R_X \leq nm + \frac{n(n + 1)}{2},$$

as one easily verifies: the lower bound gives the case that the X_i form the first n elements of the joint sample, i.e., are all lower than the Y_j, whereas the upper bound gives the case that the X_i are all greater than the Y_j.

We then form the respective difference of the actual rank-sum from the upper bound:

$$U_X = nm + \frac{n(n + 1)}{2} - R_X \text{ and } U_Y = nm + \frac{m(m + 1)}{2} - R_Y,$$

and use the minimum of these two differences as our test statistic

$$U := \min(U_X, U_Y).$$

For small n and m, the null-distribution $\mathbb{P}(U = u | H_0)$ can be tabulated by exhaustively computing all cases and counting. For large n and m, the null-distribution is very close to a normal distribution and it suffices to compute its mean and variance. Provided the null hypothesis H_0 of equal location is true, we expect the ordered X sample to be uniformly dispersed in the ordered Z sample and thus

$$\mathbb{E}(R_X) = \frac{n}{n + m}(R_X + R_Y) = \frac{n(n + m + 1)}{2},$$

in which case the variance of the rank-sum is

$$\text{Var}(R_X) = \frac{nm(n + m + 1)}{12},$$

and similarly for R_Y. The desired expectation and variance for U are then easily computed.

t-or Wilcoxon test? The *t*-test is slightly more sensitive to false positives than the Wilcoxon-test for normally distributed data, but this advantage decreases rapidly as the data deviates from normality. The Wilcoxon-test performs much better on non-normal data and is available in as many variants (one- and two-sided, multidimensional, paired observations, etc.). The Wilcoxon-test is also more conservative: if we reject using this test, we would also always reject using a *t*-test. We can therefore almost always use the Wilcoxon-test, unless we are very sure that the data is normally distributed, the variances of the two samples are very different, or we explicitly want to test the mean(s).

3.4.4 Testing Multinomial Probabilities: Pearson's χ^2

For multinomial data, like the nucleotide counts in a sequence of length n, we might want to test whether the probabilities for each category follow a particular distribution, given by the probabilities $(p_1^0, \ldots, p_s^0)$. For example, one might want to test the hypothesis that the nucleotide frequencies in the sequence are all equal by testing the null hypothesis

$$H_0 : (p_A, p_C, p_G, p_T) = (p_A^0, p_C^0, p_G^0, p_T^0) = (1/4, 1/4, 1/4, 1/4)$$

against the alternative

$$H_1 : (p_A, p_C, p_G, p_T) \neq (1/4, 1/4, 1/4, 1/4).$$

In contrast to previous examples, we test all probabilities simultaneously. *Pearson's* χ^2-*test* compares the expected number of counts in each category to the observed count x_i. The expected count under the null hypothesis is $\mathbb{E}(X_i) = np_i^0$. The χ^2-test statistic is then given by the sum of normalized differences

$$T = \sum_{i=1}^{s} \frac{(X_i - np_i^0)^2}{np_i^0}$$

and has a $\chi^2(s-1)$ distribution under the null hypothesis.

Example 28 Recall that Gregor Mendel studied peas in order to find the laws of inheritance. More specifically, he cross-bred peas and observed counts for two features, namely round/wrinkled and yellow/green, leading to four categories which we abbreviate as ry,rg,wy,wg, respectively. The theory of inheritance leads to the prediction that the frequencies for these categories should be

$$(p_{ry}^0, p_{wy}^0, p_{rg}^0, p_{wg}^0) = (9/16, 3/16, 3/16, 1/16).$$

In his original publication [1], Mendel studied $n = 556$ peas and observed the counts $x = (315, 101, 108, 32)$. This leads to a value of $t = 0.47$ for the test statistic. Using the χ^2-distribution with 3 degrees of freedom, the critical value for a test level of $\alpha = 0.05$ is given by the 0.95-quantile $\chi^2(3, 0.95) = 7.815$, and we do not reject the null hypothesis. Indeed, the p-value for this data is 0.95. As we discussed in Sect. 3.2, however, this does *not* necessarily mean that we have evidence in favor of H_0.

3.4.5 Testing Goodness-of-Fit

The χ^2-test can also be used as a *goodness-of-fit test*. This type of test is used for example to check whether some data is in agreement with given predicted values from a model. In the above example of Mendel's peas, the model of inheritance suggests a certain number of observations in each category, and the test compares this predicted numbers with the observed ones.

Let us assume that a model predicts that the results follow a certain distribution with density function $f(x; \theta)$. The l parameter(s) θ are not known. As an example, we might predict that the data is normally distributed, in which case $\theta = (\mu, \sigma^2)$ are the $l = 2$ unknown parameters.

For sample data $x_1, \ldots, x_n$, the probability to see each particular sample point x_i is zero for a continuous distribution. The main idea is thus to discretize the result by splitting the range of possible values into s non-overlapping intervals and count the number of observations in each interval. With I_j the jth such interval and some fixed parameters θ,

$$p_j(\theta) = \int_{I_j} f(x; \theta) dx$$

is the predicted probability to see an observation in this interval and we would therefore expect to see $np_j(\theta)$ observations using this parameter value.

We can now compare this expected number of observations with the observed number using the test statistics

$$T = \sum_{i=1}^{s} \frac{(N_j - np_j(\theta))^2}{np_j(\theta)},$$

which has a χ^2-distribution with $s - 1 - l$ degrees of freedom.

We are left with finding a general way to estimate the parameters θ. For reasons that cannot be properly explained here, the MLE is not a good choice, as it does not necessarily lead to a known (let alone χ^2) distribution of T under the null hypothesis. Instead, we estimate the parameters such that they maximize the objective function

$$Q(\theta) = \prod_{j=1}^{s} p_j(\theta)^{N_j},$$

which then leads to the desired χ^2-distribution of the test statistics.

Again, absence of evidence is not evidence of absence, and if the data does not give evidence to reject H_0, we cannot conclude that the hypothesis is actually correct. This is a major drawback of goodness-of-fit testing: We can only use it to check if the model could potentially explain the data, but we cannot rule out that there are other models that might fit as good. As the alternative is two-sided and composite, we also cannot flip the hypothesis, as we would need to know the distribution of T under this two-sided composite hypothesis.

3.5 Sensitivity and Specificity

In any hypothesis testing procedure, there are two types of errors that occur due to the fact that the test statistic is a random variable. There is the possibility that although H_0 is true, we observe many unusual values in the data just by chance, leading to an incorrect rejection of H_0. This is called a *false positive* or a *type-I error*. On the other hand, there is also the possibility that H_0 is false, but again the sample values suggest that it is correct, so we would incorrectly not reject H_0, which is called a *false negative* or *type-II error*. Correctly rejecting or not rejecting H_0 is called a *true positive* and *true negative*, respectively. An example for type-I and type-II errors is already given in Fig. 3.2, where we tested the mean of a normal random sample with known variance. The four possible outcomes of a hypothesis test are given in the following table:

	H_0 true	H_0 false
dont't reject H_0	true negative (TN), specificity $1 - \alpha$	false negative (FN), type-II error (β)
reject H_0	false positive (FP), type-I error (α)	true positive (TP), sensitivity $1 - \beta$

The probability $1 - \beta$ to not make a type-II error is often referred to as the *power* of the test; it is a function of the true value θ of the tested parameter. Formally, the *power function* $\eta(\theta)$ is the probability that the test statistic takes a value in the rejection region, provided that H_1 is true:

$$\eta(\theta) := 1 - \beta(\theta) = \mathbb{P}(\hat{\theta}_n \in \mathscr{R}_\alpha | H_1).$$

The power of a test is also called its *sensitivity*, as it gives the probability to correctly reject the null hypothesis if the alternative is true and therefore describes how sensitive the test is to the alternative. In addition, the probability $1 - \alpha$ of not making a type-I error, and therefore correctly not rejecting H_0 when it is true, is called the *specificity* of the test, as it describes how good the test can identify H_0 among the alternatives. Choosing a test level α therefore prescribes a fixed specificity for the test.

Specificity and sensitivity are adversaries: making one of them very high usually reduces the other. Take the following test as an example: the null hypothesis is always accepted, no matter how the data look like. Clearly, this test is very specific: it always correctly detects the null hypothesis if it is true. On the other hand, it never correctly

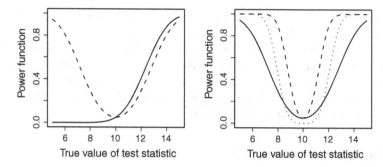

Fig. 3.4 Power functions $\eta(\mu)$ for true mean $\mu_0 = 10$ and variance $\sigma^2 = 40$. Left: One-sided H_1 : $\mu > \mu_0$ (*solid line*) and two-sided $H_1 : \mu \neq \mu_0$ alternatives (*dashed line*) for $n = 20$ and $\alpha = 0.05$. Right: two-sided alternative for $n = 20$ and $\alpha = 0.05$ (*dashed black line*), $n = 100$ and $\alpha = 0.05$ (*dashed line*), and $n = 20$ and $\alpha = 0.001$ (*dotted line*)

detects the alternative and thus has very low sensitivity. Indeed the specificity is one, the maximal possible value, while the sensitivity is zero, the minimal possible value. Always rejecting the null hypothesis gives the inverse picture.

Example 29 In Sect. 3.3.1, we tested whether the mean of a normal sample was equal to a given value. The power of this test is $\eta(\mu) = 0.882$ for $\mu = 15$ and $\eta(\mu) = 1$ for $\mu = 25$ (Fig. 3.2). The power function is

$$\eta(\mu) := 1 - \beta(\mu) = \mathbb{P}(\bar{X} > c|H_1),$$

where μ is the correct parameter value under H_1. The power is lowest if the true parameter of the alternative is close to the assumed value of the null hypothesis and it is difficult to distinguish data produced under either hypothesis. The larger the difference, the higher the power. For a difference of true and estimated parameter values $\mu - \mu_0 > 5$, the two-sided test reliably detects the alternative. The one-sided test has very low power for true values smaller than μ_0, as it does not test against these values. Almost none of these values would lead to a test statistic inside the rejection region, so the test will not reject H_0. This is correct: the one-sided alternative does not provide a better explanation of the data than the null hypothesis in this case.

We compute the power function of the one-sided test as $\eta(\mu) = 1 - \Phi(c; \mu, \sigma^2)$, where again $c = \mu + z_{1-\alpha}\sigma/\sqrt{n}$ is the critical value at the given test level. The power function for the two-sided alternative is $\eta(\mu) = 1 - (\Phi(c_h; \mu, \sigma^2) - \Phi(c_l; \mu, \sigma^2))$, where $c_l = \mu + z_{\alpha/2}\sigma/\sqrt{n}$ and $c_h = \mu + z_{1-\alpha/2}\sigma/\sqrt{n}$ are the low and high critical value, respectively. The resulting functions are given in Fig. 3.4 (*left*) for the one-sided alternative $H_1 : \mu > \mu_0$ (*solid line*) and for the two-sided alternative $H_1 : \mu \neq \mu_0$ (*dashed line*).

For a larger sample size of $n = 100$, the power of the test improves, as shown by the dashed line in Fig. 3.4 (*right*). The power function gets narrower, meaning that the test has better sensitivity closer to the value of H_0, and can thus better distinguish H_0 and H_1 in this range. Decreasing the test level to $\alpha = 0.001$ (at sample size

$n = 20$) makes the alternative more difficult to distinguish for values near μ_0, but much better further away (*dotted line*). Note that for $\mu = \mu_0$, the power function always takes value $\eta(\mu_0) = \alpha$.

3.6 Multiple Testing

So far, we always assumed that we are given one or two samples and perform one test on these samples. Many measurement techniques, however, generate massive amounts of data on which thousands of tests are performed simultaneously. In biology, the microarray allows to measure thousands of genes from the same biological sample, and differences in gene expression are tested for each individual gene. The genome of the fruit-fly, for example, has around 14,000 genes, which are all measured on one array. Assuming we test for differences in gene expression using Wilcoxon tests at a level of $\alpha = 0.05$, we would already expect to see $14,000 \times 0.05 = 700$ false positives, i.e., tests which claim that there is a significant difference between control and experiment, when in fact the difference is just by chance more extreme than expected. Because each of these 700 test results would lead to time-consuming and expensive follow-up experiments, we need to think about techniques that would allow us to deal with multiple tests in a useful way.

General Setting. Let us assume that we perform k tests simultaneously. Let V be the number of false positives, U the number of true positives, and S, T the number of true and false negatives, respectively, with k_0 correct and $k - k_0$ incorrect null-hypotheses. Importantly, we do not know k_0, but can of course observe the constant k and the realization r of R, the number of rejected hypotheses.

	H_0 true	H_0 false	
don't reject H_0	U (TN)	T (FN)	$k - R$
reject H_0	V (FP)	S (TP)	R
	k_0	$k - k_0$	k

There are two general strategies to cope with the problems posed by multiple testing: the *family-wise error rate (FWER)* tries to correct the individual test levels α such that an overall test level of α^* is achieved. Basically, these approaches try to calculate new test levels such that the chance of even one false positive is smaller than α^* and thus

$$\text{FWE} = \mathbb{P}(V > 0) \le 1 - (1 - \alpha)^k = \alpha^*.$$

One such approach is the *Bonferroni-correction*, discussed below in Sect. 3.6.1. This approach works well if the number of tests is comparatively small.

More recently, Benjamini and Hochberg introduced the concept of a *false-discovery-rate (FDR)*, which works remarkably well even for a large number of tests. We will discuss the details in Sect. 3.6.2. In essence, the FDR is the expected *false discovery ratio* of false and all positives:

$$FDR = \mathbb{E}\left(\frac{V}{R}\right) = \mathbb{E}\left(\frac{V}{S+V}\right).$$

This method explicitly allows a certain number of false positives to occur and aims at controlling the fraction of false over all positives by recalibrating the individual p-values.

3.6.1 Bonferroni-Correction

Provided we are only interested in performing a small number of tests on the data, we can use the conservative *Bonferroni-correction*. This correction implements a strategy to control the family-wise error rate. Here is the idea: let F_i be the event that hypothesis i is a false positive (it is rejected although it is actually true). The probability to have *at least one* such false positive in k tests is then

$$\mathbb{P}(V > 0) = \mathbb{P}\left(\bigcup_{i=1}^{k} F_i\right) \leq \sum_{i=1}^{k} \mathbb{P}(F_i) = \sum_{i=1}^{k} \alpha = k\alpha = \alpha^*.$$

To guarantee an overall prescribed test level of α^*, we therefore perform each individual test at level α^*/k and reject the ith null hypothesis if its p-value p_i is smaller, i.e., if

$$p_i < \frac{\alpha^*}{k}.$$

The Bonferroni-correction is very conservative as it tries to bring the overall probability of even one false positive down to α^*. Additionally, the inequality compares the true probability of the F_i to the case that the F_i are all independent, and does not try to capture the dependencies. This yields the new individual test level of α^*/k, which in many cases is much lower than would be required. For the introductory microarray example, we have $k = 14,000$ individual tests. For an overall false positive probability of $\alpha^* = 0.05$, we thus need an individual test level of $\alpha^*/k = 0.05/14,000 \approx 4e-06$, which is unrealistic to yield any meaningful results.

3.6.2 False-Discovery-Rate (FDR)

Instead of correcting the test levels such that the overall false positive probability is kept below a given threshold α^*, we can try to explicitly allow false positives to occur, but to control their expected fraction among all positives. This *false discovery rate (FDR)* is given by $FDR = \mathbb{E}(V/R)$. Again, the number of tests k is known, and the number of rejected hypotheses R is a random variable whose realization r can be observed. On the other hand, the number of false positives V is also a random variable, but its realization can not be observed. Intuitively, if we would pick one of the rejected hypotheses at random, the FDR can be interpreted as the expected chance that this hypothesis was falsely rejected. For 100 rejected hypotheses, an FDR of 0.05 would also mean that we expect that $100 \times 0.05 = 5$ of these are false positives. To achieve a certain FDR in a concrete situation, we need to choose the number of rejections such that the prescribed FDR is reached; we can do this by appropriately adjusting the p-value for which to reject.

Benjamini-Hochberg procedure. We would like to have strategy that guarantees a proportion of false positives of at most q^* among all rejected hypotheses. For this, we calculate at which p-value to reject a hypothesis such that the FDR stays below this desired threshold q^* as follows: we expect $\mathbb{E}(V) = \alpha k$ false positives in k tests for a given test level α. For a given set of data, the number of null hypotheses rejected at this level is $r(\alpha)$, a realization of R. The *Benjamini-Hochberg procedure* computes this number $r(\alpha)$ such that the maximal number of hypotheses are rejected while still keeping the expected proportion of false positives below the given threshold q^*, thus

$$\mathbb{E}\left(\frac{V}{R}\right) = \frac{\alpha k}{r(\alpha)} \leq q^*.$$

Let again p_i be the p-value of the ith hypothesis test and consider the ordered p-values $p_{(1)} \leq \cdots \leq p_{(k)}$. We then compute the largest index l such that

$$p_{(i)} \leq \frac{i}{k}q^*$$

for all $(i) < l$. The values $q_i = \frac{i}{k}q^*$ are sometimes called the q-values. One can show that if we reject those null hypotheses for which $p_i \leq q_l = \frac{l}{k}q^*$,

$$\text{FDR} \leq \frac{k_0}{k}q^* \leq q^*,$$

which guarantees the desired proportion of false positives.

Comparing p-values and q-values. Despite some similarities, p-values and q-values have some fundamental differences. The p-value gives the smallest test level at which not to reject and thus needs to be correct and exact to assess the data. On the other hand, q^* is a threshold for an expected ratio, so the actual ratio might be higher. It serves more as a "calling" tool that filters out uninteresting test results from a large number of performed tests. A proper analysis would then further investigate the remaining candidates, so it is usually not problematic if the desired q^* is not exactly achieved in the actual study.

Example 30 Let us consider the scenario that $k = 10$ individual tests were performed on data and that their ordered p-values $p_{(i)}$ are

$$0.00017, 0.003, 0.0071, 0.0107, 0.014, 0.32, 0.4, 0.54, 0.58, 0.98.$$

For an overall test level of $\alpha^* = 0.05$, the Bonferroni correction then requires individual test levels of $\alpha = \alpha^*/k = 0.005$ and we would reject the first 2 null hypotheses. On the other hand, we could decide to allow an expected fraction of $q^* = 0.05$ false positives among all rejected hypotheses. Using the Benjamini-Hochberg method, we compute the corresponding q-values to be

$$0.005, 0.01, 0.015, 0.02, 0.025, 0.03, 0.035, 0.04, 0.045, 0.05,$$

and $p_{(5)} = 0.014 < 0.025 = q_5$ whereas $p_{(6)} = 0.32 > 0.03 = q_6$; we would consequently be able to reject the first 5 null hypotheses.

3.7 Combining Results of Multiple Experiments

Let us imagine that three groups independently did a particular experiment and each group performed the same test on their data. The reported p-values are 0.08, 0.06, and 0.07, respectively, none of them significant at the $\alpha = 0.05$ level. However, we might argue that it seems unlikely that all three tests are so close to the 0.05-level just by chance and that combined, the three tests actually give significant evidence to reject the null hypothesis.

We can invoke the following argument to justify this idea: let t_i be the value of the test statistic T_i of test i, leading to a p-value of p_i, and let us again assume k independent tests. If the null hypothesis were true in all cases, we can ask for the joint probability of simultaneously observing the given values of the test statistics:

$$\mathbb{P}(T_1 > t_1, \ldots, T_k > t_k | H_0) = \prod_{i=1}^{k} \mathbb{P}(T_i > t_i | H_0),$$

which corresponds to asking for the probability that the observed p-values occur under H_0.

Let P_i be the p-value of the ith test, treated as a random variable. It can be shown that the P_i are uniformly distributed on [0,1] under H_0 and thus each p-value is equally likely if the null hypothesis is correct. However, the product of uniform random variables is itself not uniform, so we need to calculate the corresponding distribution. A simple trick comes to the rescue: the logarithm of a uniform random variable U, scaled by (-2), has a χ^2-distribution with two degrees of freedom:

$$-2\log(U) \sim \chi^2(2),$$

and we know from Sect. 1.4 that the sum of χ^2-variables still has a χ^2-distribution, with corresponding degrees of freedom:

$$Q = -2 \sum_{i=1}^{k} \log(P_i) \sim \chi^2(2k).$$

This allows us to combine p-values from different experiments, provided the same test was used in each experiment. We compute the realization q of Q from the observed p-values and reject the null hypothesis if $q > \chi^2_{1-\alpha}(2k)$.

Example 31 For the p-values 0.08, 0.06, and 0.07, we compute the value

$$q = -2 \times (\log(0.08) + \log(0.06) + \log(0.07)) = 15.9968$$

for the test statistic Q. With $k = 3$, this statistic has a $\chi^2(6)$-distribution, and the overall P-value is thus $p = \mathbb{P}(Q > q | H_0) \approx 0.0138$. While each individual result does not give evidence against the null hypothesis, the combination of the three experiments shows significant evidence that the null hypothesis is false.

3.8 Summary

To test a property of a distribution, we formulate two hypotheses—the null hypothesis H_0 and the alternative hypothesis H_1—,such that the null hypothesis represents the "status quo". We then compute the value for a test statistic T from a random sample; the distribution of T under the null hypothesis allows us to compute the p-value—the probability of a false rejection. The smaller the p-value, the less likely H_0 is true and we reject it if the p-value is below a prescribed test level α. However, we can not prove the correctness of a null hypothesis and the p-value is not the probability that H_0 is correct.

Before choosing a test statistic, it is often worthwhile to check whether robust alternatives are available, such as the Wilcoxon-test to replace a classic t-test.

The sensitivity and specificity of a test describe the probabilities to correctly reject or not reject the null hypothesis. They depend on the test statistic, the two hypotheses, but also on the sample size.

When preforming several tests simultaneously, we need to recalibrate the p-values to correct for multiple testing, which we can do either by the Bonferroni-method, which controls the probability to get even one false positive, or using the false discovery rate approach, which allows a prescribed fraction of false positives among all rejected hypotheses.

Reference

1. Mendel, G.: Versuche über Pflanzenhybriden. Verhandlungen des naturforschenden Vereines in Brünn **IV**, 3–47 (1866)

Chapter 4
Regression

Abstract Regression analysis describes the influence of covariates on a response variable. Two regression models are discussed: linear regression on one or several covariates and analysis-of-variance. Methods for estimating the respective model parameters and hypothesis tests for eliminating non-significant covariates are presented.

Keywords Linear regression · Model reduction · ANOVA

All models are wrong but some are useful

George E. P. Box

4.1 Introduction

Regression analysis aims at studying the influence of one or more *covariates X* on a *response Y*. We only discuss *parametric regression*, where we know the functional relation between covariates and response, and try to identify the correct parameter(s) of this function. The *regression function* is then defined as the expected value conditioned on the values of the covariates:

$$r(x; \theta) = \mathbb{E}(Y|X = x) = \int y f(y|x; \theta) \mathrm{d}y,$$

where $f(y|x; \theta)$ is the conditional probability density of $Y|X$ with parameters θ. Once we know the parameters, we can predict the average value for the response for any given values of the covariates by the regression function. For estimating the parameters from given data, we assume that we have n samples

$$(y_1, x_{1,1}, x_{1,2}, \ldots, x_{1,m}), \ldots, (y_n, x_{n,1}, x_{n,2}, \ldots, x_{n,m}),$$

H.-M. Kaltenbach, *A Concise Guide to Statistics*, SpringerBriefs in Statistics,
DOI: 10.1007/978-3-642-23502-3_4, © Hans-Michael Kaltenbach 2012

where y_i is the value of the response variable in the ith measurement and $x_{i,j}$ is the value of the jth covariate for that measurement. Regression analysis assumes that the values of the covariates $x_{i,j}$ are known exactly. In contrast, the observed values of the response y_i are subject to error and an *error model* is used to described their distribution around the true value. The assumed relation of covariates and response is then

$$Y = r(x; \theta) + \varepsilon,$$

where ε is a random error term.

Example 32 Let us consider the problem of finding the relation between the dry weight and height of a plant. We may claim that the dry weight increases linearly with the height of the plant. Using the height as a covariate x and the dry weight as the response y, we can use the following linear regression model to describe this relation:

$$Y = \beta_0 + \beta_1 x + \varepsilon.$$

Here, the parameter β_0 is the dry weight of a plant with height zero, and β_1 describes how much more dry weight we get per increase in height. We implicitly assume that the height can be measured without error, but the measured weight spreads around the true value by an error ε. The first task is then to measure the weight and height of n plants, yielding the data (y_1, x_1) to (y_n, x_n). From this data, we would then try to find the correct parameter values for β_0 and β_1. Once these are established, we can predict the dry weight from the height of any new plant.

4.2 Classes of Regression Problems

Depending on the type of covariates and response, we can distinguish several classes of regression problems. The two main types are *metric* variables, which are any kind of (continuous) numbers, and *categorial* variables, which describe membership in distinct classes. Examples for the first type are measurements of length, (discrete) counts, and waiting times, for the second type categories such as male/female. Categories can sometimes additionally have an order such as high > middle > low, and variables are then called *ordinal*.

   If both response and covariates are metric, we are in the setting usually called regression, and we can further distinguish linear from nonlinear regression, depending on the claimed functional relation $r()$. Linear regression is the typical first example of regression methods and will be covered in detail in Sect. 4.3 for a single covariate. If several covariates are involved, powerful methods can be applied to reduce the model and identify those covariates which have a significant influence on the response. The required methods for estimation and hypothesis testing are covered in Sect. 4.4.

Regression of a metric response on categorial covariates requires Analysis-of-Variance (ANOVA). The impact of treatment (no drug/drug A/drug B) on the recovery time of a patient is an example. ANOVA can be seen as an extension of t-tests to more than two means; we discuss ANOVA in Sect. 4.5. After presenting the estimators for the ANOVA model parameters, we also develop hypothesis tests to investigate the influence of combinations of groups on the response variable.

4.3 Linear Regression: One Covariate

We start by discussing linear regression with one covariate. This is the workhorse in regression analysis; it is widely applicable in practice and many other methods can be derived as variants and extensions.

4.3.1 Problem Statement

Linear regression with one covariate assumes a regression function of the form

$$Y = \beta_0 + \beta_1 X + \varepsilon,$$

where Y is the metric response to the metric covariate X. The parameters (in linear regression traditionally called β) of this family of regression functions are the intercept β_0 and the slope β_1 of the (x, y)-line.

It is the error term ε that prevents us from observing the correct response directly, and makes Y a random variable. We assume the error to have zero mean, so it does not introduce a bias in the analysis. We further assume that it has constant (but unknown) variance σ^2, independent of the value x of the covariate; this is called *homoscedacity*:

$$\mathbb{E}(\varepsilon|X = x) = 0$$
$$\mathrm{Var}(\varepsilon|X = x) = \sigma^2.$$

If the variance of the error does depend on the value x, we call this *heteroscedacity*. For some of the analyses, we do not need to assume a particular distribution of ε, but for more sophisticated analyses, we often assume that the error has a normal distribution. Section 4.3.3 is devoted to methods for checking these assumptions on the error structure.

4.3.2 Parameter Estimation

Without assuming any particular error distribution, we cannot apply the maximum-likelihood principle and therefore rely on a least-squares method for estimating the two parameters β_0 and β_1. Given the parameter values, the value

$$\hat{y}_i = r(x_i) = \beta_0 + \beta_1 x_i$$

is the *predicted response* to the value x_i of the covariate. We can apply least-squares estimation to find those parameter values $\hat{\beta}_0$ and $\hat{\beta}_1$ that minimize the squared differ-ence $\hat{\varepsilon}_i^2 = (y_i - \hat{y}_i)^2$ between the measured and the predicted value:

$$(\hat{\beta}_0, \hat{\beta}_1) = \mathrm{argmin}_{\beta_0, \beta_1} \sum_{i=1}^{n} \hat{\varepsilon}_i^2 = \mathrm{argmin}_{\beta_0, \beta_1} \sum_{i=1}^{n} (y_i - (\beta_0 + \beta_1 x_i))^2 .$$

The differences $\hat{\varepsilon}_i^2$ are called the *residuals* and are themselves estimates of the error ε in each sample point.

This least-squares problem always has a unique solution and we even find explicit formulas for the estimates:

$$\hat{\beta}_1 = \frac{\sum_{i=1}^{n}(x_i - \bar{x})(y_i - \bar{y})}{\sum_{i=1}^{n}(x_i - \bar{x})^2}$$

$$\hat{\beta}_0 = \bar{y} - \hat{\beta}_1 \bar{x},$$

from which we can also estimate the variance of the error by

$$\hat{\sigma}^2 = \frac{1}{n-2} \sum_{i=1}^{n} \hat{\varepsilon}_i^2,$$

using $n - 2$ degrees of freedom (one less per estimated $\hat{\beta}_i$).

Example 33 A typical example is shown in Fig. 4.1, where 10 responses were measured from a linear function $y = \beta_0 + \beta_1 x + \varepsilon$ with true parameters $\beta_0 = 2$ and $\beta_1 = 4$ and normally distributed error with variance $\sigma^2 = 40$. Using the least-squares method, the parameters are estimated as $\hat{\beta}_0 = -0.085$ and $\hat{\beta}_1 = 4.377$. The estimated standard deviation is $\hat{\sigma}^2 = 118.926$. The solid line gives the predicted responses $\hat{y}_i$ for any value x of the covariate. The residuals $\hat{\varepsilon}_i$ are then the vertical differences between this line and the actual response value y_i for a measurement, indicated by vertical dashed lines.

MLE under normality. If in addition to homoscedacity and unbiasedness, the error is normally distributed, we can also apply the maximum-likelihood approach to find the parameters β_0, β_1. Interestingly this yields the exact same estimators and thus maximum-likelihood and least-squares estimates coincide under normality of errors.

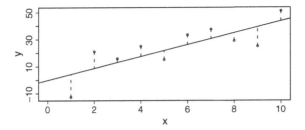

Fig. 4.1 Linear regression of 10 measurements: Fitted regression $y = \hat{\beta}_0 + \hat{\beta}_1 x$ (*solid line*), residuals $\hat{\varepsilon}_i$ (*dashed lines*) and data (y_i, x_i) (*black points*). True parameters are $\beta_0 = 2$ and $\beta_1 = 4$ with an error variance of $\sigma^2 = 40$ with estimates $\hat{\beta}_0 = -0.085$, $\hat{\beta}_1 = 4.377$, and $\hat{\sigma}^2 = 118.926$

The MLEs for the two parameters are consistent and unbiased. As MLEs, they also have an asymptotic normal distribution, so confidence intervals for the estimated parameters are given by

$$\hat{\beta}_i \pm z_{\alpha/2}\widehat{se}(\hat{\beta}_i),$$

where the estimators' standard errors $\widehat{se}(\hat{\beta}_i) = \sqrt{\widehat{Var}(\hat{\beta}_i)}$ are

$$\widehat{se}(\hat{\beta}_0) = \frac{\hat{\sigma}}{\hat{\sigma}_X \sqrt{n}} \sqrt{\frac{1}{n} \sum_{i=1}^{n} x_i^2},$$

$$\widehat{se}(\hat{\beta}_1) = \frac{\hat{\sigma}}{\hat{\sigma}_X \sqrt{n}},$$

and $\hat{\sigma}_X^2 = \frac{1}{n-1} \sum_{i=1}^{n} (x_i - \bar{x})^2$ is the dispersion of values taken for the covariate. We can even give the full covariance matrix, which contains the variance of the two estimators in the diagonal, and the covariance of them in the off-diagonals:

$$\widehat{Var}\begin{pmatrix} \hat{\beta}_0 \\ \hat{\beta}_1 \end{pmatrix} = \frac{\hat{\sigma}^2}{\hat{\sigma}_X^2 n} \begin{pmatrix} \frac{1}{n} \sum_{i=1}^{n} x_i^2 & -\bar{x} \\ -\bar{x} & 1 \end{pmatrix}.$$

Prediction intervals. Once the parameters are estimated from the data, we can apply this "fitted" regression model to predict the value Y_* of the response for other values x_* of the covariate by

$$\hat{Y}_* = \hat{\beta}_0 + \hat{\beta}_1 x_*.$$

Although for given parameters this gives a particular prediction, this prediction still depends on the estimated values $\hat{\beta}_i$. Since these in turn depend on the original data used for the estimation, the prediction $\hat{Y}_*$ is still a random variable and we should compute a confidence interval for $\hat{Y}_*$ to quantify the confidence in the prediction.

This interval depends on the error ε, but also on the error in the estimates $\hat{\beta}_i$ and is given by

$$\hat{Y}_* \pm z_{\alpha/2}\hat{\zeta},$$

where the standard deviation $\hat{\zeta}$ is *not* the estimated standard deviation of the estimator, but is given by

$$\hat{\zeta}^2 = \hat{\sigma}^2 \left(\frac{\sum_{i=1}^{n}(x_i - x_*)^2}{n\sum_{i=1}^{n}(x_i - \bar{x})^2} + 1 \right).$$

This confidence interval depends on the variance of the data, but additionally gets wider, the further away the new covariate value x_* is from the original values used in the estimation of the parameters. For example, if values of the covariate in the original sample are all between $x_1 = 1$ and $x_n = 10$, an *extrapolation* by predicting the outcome for $x_* = 100$ gives a much wider confidence interval than an *interpolation* at a value $x_* = 5$.

4.3.3 Checking Assumptions

Application of standard linear regression techniques relies on two assumptions: homoscedacity of the data, i.e., constant variance independent of the covariate, and, for many conclusions, normally distributed errors. To check these assumptions, we can perform an *a posteriori* analysis of the resulting residuals $y_i - \hat{y}_i$ after estimating the parameters.

Checking homoscedacity. Homoscedacity can be assessed by plotting the residuals $\hat{\varepsilon}_i$ of the fitted model against the covariate values x_i. We then expect to see no particular pattern and points should scatter uniformly around zero. If the variance increases with the value of the covariate—one of the most common causes of heteroscedacity—a tilted 'V' pattern appears as the residuals get bigger with increasing x_i.

For 50 sample points using the same linear regression function as before, the residuals are shown in Fig. 4.2 (left). Changing the error model such that the variance increase linearly with the covariate yields the tilted 'V' pattern in Fig. 4.2 (right).

Checking normality. Assessing whether the error distribution is normal is straightforward once the model parameters are estimated. If the error distribution is normal, the resulting residuals should follow a normal distribution with mean $\mu = 0$ and the estimated variance $\hat{\sigma}^2$. We can use a normal Q–Q-plot for visual inspection. For the example above with $n = 50$ sample points, the normal Q–Q-plots of the residuals are shown in Fig. 4.3 for both homoscedacity (left) and heteroscedacity (right). In both plots, the residuals scatter around a mean of zero, and do not introduce a bias in the estimation, as expected.

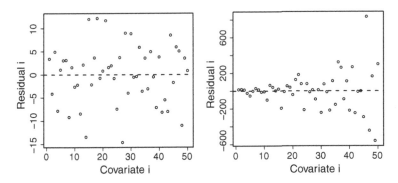

Fig. 4.2 *Left* Residuals $\hat{\varepsilon}_i$ of fitted model (points) spread around zero (*dashed line*) and show no particular pattern. *Right* Residuals show heteroscedacity and form a titled 'V' pattern as the variance increases with increasing covariate

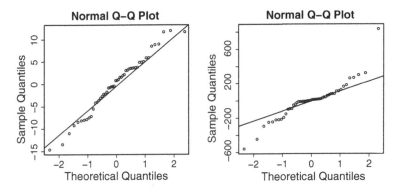

Fig. 4.3 Normal Q–Q-plot of residuals in the case of homo- (*left*) and hetero-scedacity (*right*)

4.3.4 Linear Regression Using R

R already provides all necessary functions for easily fitting linear models. For given data vectors x and y, a linear regression is fitted using the function lm(), which requires an *R formula* as input. R formulas are a very convenient way of representing complex regression problems. An example is

$$y \sim x + z,$$

which states that we want a fit of the response y on the two covariates x and z. Thus, R fits the model $Y = \beta_0 + \beta_1 X + \beta_2 Z$ by estimating the three parameters β_i. In R formulas, the arithmetic operators $+, -, *, /$ as well as exponents have special interpretations, and should not be confused with their usual meaning.

Parameter estimation. Let us consider a linear regression problem with one covariate. The covariate vector x contains the values of the covariate and the response vector y the corresponding values of the response. Then, the R command

```
model <- lm(y ~ x)
```

estimates the various parameters and yields a data-structure `model` containing all the information about the resulting linear model.

Inspection plots. The model can then be plotted using the command `plot(model)` to successively generate four plots: the residuals, the normal Q–Q-plot, the residuals on another scale, and an influence plot (see Sect. 4.4.4 for a discussion of different influence measures).

Model plot. We can also easily plot the model together with the data by first plotting the data by `plot(y ~ x)`, and then adding the estimated regression line with `abline(model)`. This was done to generate Fig. 4.1.

Prediction. Predicting new values from a model is done using the `predict()` function, which expects a model data-structure and a data-frame with the new values of the covariates. For example

```
predict(object=model, newdata=new.x, interval='prediction')
```

for two new values $x = 2.4$ and $x = 90$ yields the result

```
     fit          lwr          upr
1   12.78273    -2.671691    28.23715
2  349.02757   217.846374   480.20877
```

with the predicted values in the first column and the lower and upper value of the 0.95-prediction intervals in the second and third column.

4.3.5 On the "Linear" in Linear Regression

An important point to understand when using linear regression models is that we only need the regression function to be linear *in the parameters*. For example, the model

$$Y = \beta_0 + \beta_1 X^2$$

is a perfectly valid linear regression model, because we may simply replace the covariate X with a new covariate $Z = X^2$ to get the familiar equation. Other models can be made linear by transformation. For example, the model

$$Y = \beta_0 \exp(\beta_1 X)$$

is easily brought into a form suitable for linear regression by taking the logarithm. However, there is a caveat: if the original model has additive, normally distributed error, this error structure is also transformed by the logarithm and is no longer normal. This can cause major problems, as many of the statistics rely on normally distributed residuals.

4.4 Linear Regression: Multiple Covariates

For more than one covariate, linear regression aims at fitting a *hyperplane* through a cloud of points. Again, all values of covariates are assumed to be fixed and non-random, and only the value of the response is subject to error.

Example 34 Let us reconsider our small introductory example of studying dry weight as a function of height in plants. Instead of using only the height, we may also want to consider more variables that might have an influence on the dry weight. For example, we could study the influence of the amount of fertilizer on the weight. The model would then informally read

$$\text{dry weight} = \beta_0 + \beta_1 \text{ height} + \beta_2 \text{ fertilizer amount} + \text{error}.$$

This allows us to ask more questions on the model, for example if the fertilizer has any influence at all. If not, we could delete it from the model, which would result in a new and more simple model that is still able to sufficiently describe the dry weight. Regression analysis also allows us to explicitly take the influence of the covariates on each other into account. Here, we might consider that more fertilizer also yields higher plants, which we need to take into consideration when trying to find the most simple model that sufficiently explains the data.

4.4.1 Problem Statement

We are studying a regression problem with m covariates $X_1, \ldots, X_m$ and one response variable Y. The data are again n tuples of sample points, each with one value for each covariate and one value for the noisy measured response. The regression model is then of the form

$$Y = \beta_0 + \beta_1 X_1 + \beta_2 X_2 + \cdots + \beta_m X_m + \varepsilon$$

and might additionally contain interaction terms to capture the dependency of covariates on each other. The resulting estimation problem of n equations in m covariates can then be written as

$$\begin{pmatrix} y_1 \\ \vdots \\ y_n \end{pmatrix} = \begin{pmatrix} 1 & x_{1,1} & \cdots & x_{1,m} \\ \vdots & \vdots & & \vdots \\ 1 & x_{n,1} & \cdots & x_{n,m} \end{pmatrix} \cdot \begin{pmatrix} \beta_0 \\ \vdots \\ \beta_m \end{pmatrix} + \begin{pmatrix} \varepsilon_1 \\ \vdots \\ \varepsilon_n \end{pmatrix},$$

using matrix-vector notation. The matrix $\mathbf{X}$ containing the $x_{i,j}$ is called the *design matrix*, where the first column is the "covariate" for the constant term β_0. We again assume that each ε_i has mean zero and constant variance and that the errors are independent. For most of the statistics, we additionally require the errors to be normally distributed.

4.4.2 Parameter Estimation

We can again estimate the parameters as $\hat{\beta} = (\hat{\beta}_0, \ldots, \hat{\beta}_m)$ by minimizing the sum of squared differences

$$\hat{\beta} = \text{argmin}_\beta \sum_{i=1}^n \left(y_i - \left(\beta_0 + \beta_1 x_{i,1} + \cdots + \beta_m x_{i,m} \right) \right)^2.$$

Again, the estimates can be given in explicit form by

$$\hat{\beta} = \left(\mathbf{X}'\mathbf{X} \right)^{-1} \mathbf{X}'\mathbf{Y},$$

where $\mathbf{X}$ is the above design matrix containing the covariate values and a 1 entry in the first column and $\mathbf{Y}$ is the vector containing the n values of the response.

4.4.3 Hypothesis Testing and Model Reduction

A natural question to ask is whether we really need all the covariates to explain the measured responses, or if a smaller subset of covariates will already explain the data. This is the question for a *minimal adequate model*, which is the model with the smallest number of covariates that still explains the data reasonably well. In general, the data can always be better explained with more covariates, simply because we get more parameters to work with. However, reducing the model by eliminating one covariate and its associated parameter might lead to a new model that is almost as good as the larger model. For doing this properly, we need a way of quantifying what we mean by "almost as good". We start with a central result on decomposing the overall variation that will then naturally lead to the required statistics.

Decomposing the variation. Without considering any regression, the *total variation* in the response is

$$\text{SS}_{\text{tot}} = \sum_{i=1}^n (y_i - \bar{y})^2.$$

It is proportional to $\text{Var}(Y)$ with a factor of $(n-1)$ and is a measure of the overall dispersion of the response around its mean.

After fitting a regression model, this total variation can be decomposed into two components: the *explained variation* or *regression sum-of-squares*

$$\text{SS}_{\text{reg}} = \sum_{i=1}^n \left(\hat{y}_i - \bar{y} \right)^2,$$

which measures how much of the total variation can be explained by the fact that the measured response is actually spread around the regression line and not simply around its mean, and the *error sum-of-squares*

Fig. 4.4 (Adapted from [1])
Total variation as sum of
explained and unexplained
variation. Each difference
$y_i - \bar{y}$ of a measured to the
mean response can be
decomposed into the
difference $\hat{y}_i - \bar{y}$ of the mean
and the predicted regression
value and the difference
$y_i - \hat{y}_i$ between predicted
and measured value

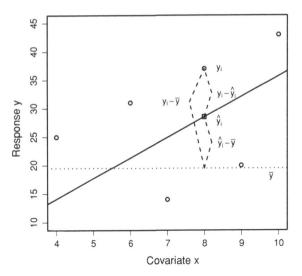

$$SS_{err} = \sum_{i=1}^{n} \left(y_i - \hat{y}_i \right)^2,$$

which gives the *unexplained variation* still left, i.e., the dispersion of the measured response values around their predicted values. Note that SS_{err} is exactly the residual sum-of-squares $\sum_i \hat{\varepsilon}_i^2$ that is minimized for estimation.

Using the regression model, the total variation can always be written as the sum of the explained and the unexplained variation:

$$SS_{tot} = SS_{reg} + SS_{err},$$

which is also demonstrated in Fig. 4.4.

The variance can be recovered by dividing a variation by its corresponding degrees of freedom, which are $SS_{tot} : n - 1$, $SS_{reg} : m$, and $SS_{err} : n - m - 1$.

Varying the parameters β_i of the regression function does not change the *measured* response values, so the total variation SS_{tot} remains the same. However, we will alter the *predicted* response values and thus the contributions of the explained and unexplained variations to the total variation. A "good" set of parameters will have a large SS_{reg}, so a lot of the total variation is explained by the fact that the response spreads around the regression function rather than its mean. The remaining unexplained variation caused by this spread around the regression function is minimized in this case.

We can exploit this decomposition of the total variation in two ways: First, it gives the *coefficient of determination* $R^2 = SS_{reg}/SS_{tot}$, which is the proportion of explained to total variation. Consider using the model $Y = \beta_0 + \varepsilon$ with no covariates, leading to the fit $\hat{\beta}_0 = \bar{y}$ with constant predicted response. The coefficient of determination is zero in this case and the model cannot explain any of the deviation of measured y_i from their mean. For a perfect linear fit with no measurement error, the coefficient is one, as the data is completely explained by the model. For a linear regression using a single covariate, the coefficient of determination is identical to the *Pearson's correlation coefficient* (see Sect. 1.6.4), given by

$$R^2 = \frac{\text{Cov}(X, Y)}{\sigma_X \sigma_Y}.$$

In addition to the coefficient of determination, we can also use the decomposition to compare models with a different number of covariates. For normally distributed errors, the various sum-of-squares all have χ^2-distributions with appropriate degrees of freedom. Thus, the quotient

$$F = \frac{\text{SS}_{\text{reg}}/m}{\text{SS}_{\text{err}}/(n - m - 1)}$$

of the explained versus the unexplained variation has an $F(m, n-m-1)$-distribution (see Sect. 1.4). The larger this value becomes, the better the regression explains the data.

Do we need any covariate? Now that we have worked out a way to quantify how good a regression explains the data, we can start asking statistical questions on the relevance of the various covariates for this explanation. The boldest question is to ask whether the regression actually explains the data at all. For this, we define the *null model* $Y = \beta_0 + \varepsilon$ which in essence states that the data can be explained by the spread around its mean alone. We then compare this null model to the *full model* $Y = \beta_0 + \sum_j \beta_j X_j + \varepsilon$ including all covariates. This comparison requires to test the hypothesis

$$H_0 : \beta_1 = \cdots = \beta_m = 0$$

that it suffices to only consider β_0 (i.e., the null model) estimated as $\hat{\beta}_0 = \bar{y}$ to describe the data and the covariates thus have no relation to the response. With

$$F = \frac{\text{SS}_{\text{reg}}/m}{\text{SS}_{\text{err}}/(n - m - 1)}$$

as our test statistic, we reject this null hypothesis if F exceeds the corresponding quantile of the F-distribution: $F > F_{1-\alpha}(m, n - m - 1)$.

This hypothesis test can serve as a sanity check: if we do not find evidence to reject this hypothesis, the proposed model is not able to explain the data and none of the covariates has a significant (linear) relation to the response.

Testing subsets of covariates. The same ideas allow us to check if a *reduced model*, using only a subset of the covariates, already provides a sufficient fit to the data. More specifically, we want to test the hypothesis

$$H_0 : \beta_{k+1} = \cdots = \beta_m = 0$$

that only the first k covariates are needed and the remaining $m - k$ covariates do not provide any more explanation of the observed data. We only consider the first covariates simply to avoid clumsy notation; clearly, the exact same method works for any subset of covariates by simply re-ordering them.

Let us denote by $SS_{reg}(k)$ the explained variation of the reduced model, with only the first k covariates present, and similar notation for the remaining variables. The special case $SS_{reg}(m) \equiv SS_{reg}$ then denotes the previously explained variation of the full model.

The test statistic

$$F_k = \frac{\left(SS_{reg}(m) - SS_{reg}(k)\right)/(m - k)}{SS_{err}/(n - m - 1)}$$

has a $F(m - k, n - m - 1)$ distribution and we can reject the null hypothesis at the level α if $F_k > F_{1-\alpha}(m - k, n - m - 1)$. If we can reject H_0, we conclude that the $m - k$ covariates not contained in the reduced model do not significantly contribute to the explanation of the data. Importantly, the term "significantly" is well-defined in this context. By setting $k = 0$, we re-derive the previous hypothesis that we do not need any covariate.

Model reduction. By exhaustively testing all possible reduced models, we can compute a minimal adequate model; it has the smallest number of covariates such that adding any of the other covariates does not significantly increase the model's fit. For m covariates, there are 2^m different models from subsets of the covariates. For larger models, one therefore retreats to iterative procedures for finding a minimal adequate model. The two simplest procedures either start with the full model and iteratively discard one covariate at a time, or start with the empty model and iteratively add one covariate. The order in which this is done may however impact the result, especially if the covariates influence each other.

Example 35 Consider the following experiment: we want to investigate the influence of the concentration x_1, x_2, x_3 of three different chemicals on the production rate y of a particular other chemical. We use a regression model that takes y as the response to various combinations of the three concentrations, each taken as a covariate. The linear regression model assumes that the response is the results of adding the three covariates with different scaling factors. We aim at finding the minimal adequate linear model to describe the response. We first try to get a visual impression of the data by investigating all pairwise scatter plots in Fig. 4.5. In this plot, we observe a number of relations: first, the three covariates do not seem to interact with each other, i.e., they appear to be independent. Second, the most pronounced influence on y seems to be from x_3, and it appears to be slightly curved. Moreover, there appears to be a correlation between response and x_1, and only a weak response to x_2. We therefore start with a full model that contains the three individual covariates together with their squares (to capture the potential curvature), and no interaction terms. The following R command will compute the parameter estimation for this model:

```
m <- lm(y ~ x1 + x2 + x3 + I(x1^2) + I(x2^2) + I(x3^2), data = d)
```

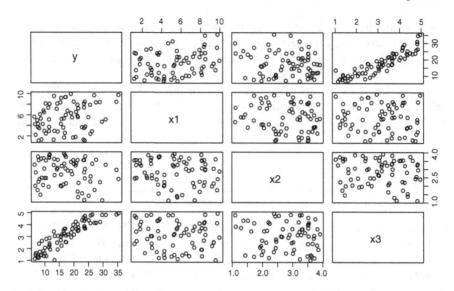

Fig. 4.5 All pairwise scatter plots of response y and covariates x_1 to x_3

The function $\texttt{I()}$ tells R to interpret its content as an arithmetic expression, rather than an R formula. This command will fit the model

$$Y = \beta_0 + \beta_1 X_1 + \beta_2 X_2 + \beta_3 X_3 + \beta_4 X_1^2 + \beta_5 X_2^2 + \beta_6 X_3^2.$$

The resulting estimates are shown using $\texttt{summary(m)}$.

```
Call:
lm(formula = y ~ x1 + x2 + x3 + I(x1^2) + I(x2^2) + I(x3^2), data = d)
```

Residuals:

Min	1Q	Median	3Q	Max
−2.05561	−0.58005	−0.08151	0.77322	1.66987

Coefficients:

	Estimate	Std. Error	t value	Pr(> |t|)	
(Intercept)	0.791207	1.827610	0.433	0.667	
x1	0.984675	0.224661	4.383	4.52e − 05	***
x2	0.517541	1.117399	0.463	0.645	
x3	−0.169954	0.570742	−0.298	0.767	
I(x1^2)	0.003262	0.020030	0.163	0.871	
I(x2^2)	−0.080277	0.210408	−0.382	0.704	
I(x3^2)	1.014840	0.093811	10.818	5.33e − 16	***

```
---
Signif. codes: 0 '***' 0.001 '**' 0.01 '*' 0.05 '.' 0.1 ' ' 1

Residual standard error: 0.9389 on 63 degrees of freedom
Multiple R-squared: 0.9844,        Adjusted R-squared: 0.9829
F-statistic: 663 on 6 and 63 DF, p-value: < 2.2e-16
```

In this summary, R states the fitted model and a summary of the distribution of the residuals, and then returns the estimated value and the standard deviation for each parameter, as well as a test statistic and corresponding p-value on the significance of this parameter. These statistics are t-distributed, and test the null hypothesis $H_0 : \beta_i = 0$ that the corresponding covariate is not needed; recall from Sect. 1.4 that $F(1, m) = t^2(m)$. In this full model, x_3 is not significant and has a high p-value, making it a good candidate for model reduction, but its square is highly significant. Overall, a very good fit was found, indicated by an R^2-value of 0.9844.

From this first result, we start reducing the model by deleting x_3 (but not its square) using the update() function, which takes the fitted model and an update to the original formula to compute a new model. The command

```
m2 <- update(m, ˜. − x3)
```

fits this new model, where the dot denotes the old formula, from which parts are discarded, resulting in

```
Call:
lm(formula = y ˜ x1 + x2 + I(x1^2) + I(x2^2) + I(x3^2), data = d)

Residuals:
Min            1Q            Median    3Q        Max
-2.0659        -0.6043       -0.1029   0.7711    1.6468

Coefficients:
                Estimate    Std. Error   t value   Pr(> |t|)
(Intercept)     0.583431    1.677100     0.348     0.729
x1              0.986668    0.222957     4.425     3.83e − 05 * **
x2              0.501293    1.108091     0.452     0.653
I(x1^2)         0.003054    0.019874     0.154     0.878
I(x2^2)        -0.077590    0.208712    -0.372     0.711
I(x3^2)         0.987357    0.016691     59.155    ≤ 2e − 16 * **
---
Signif. codes: 0 '***' 0.001 '**' 0.01 '*' 0.05 '.' 0.1 ' ' 1

Residual standard error: 0.9322 on 64 degrees of freedom
Multiple R-squared: 0.9844,            Adjusted R-squared: 0.9832
F-statistic: 807.1 on 5 and 64 DF, p-value: < 2.2e-16
```

Using the anova() function, we can compare the first and reduced model. This function will compute exactly the F-test described above and test the hypothesis $H_0 : \beta_3 = 0$ that x_3 is not significant and can be discarded without significantly changing the ability of the model to explain the data. The call

$$\text{anova(m, m2)}$$

yields the following result:

Analysis of Variance Table

```
Model 1 : y ~ x1 + x2 + x3 + I(x1^2) + I(x2^2) + I(x3^2)
Model 2 : y ~ x1 + x2 + I(x1^2) + I(x2^2) + I(x3^2)
     Res.Df      RSS        Df    Sum of Sq     F  Pr(> F)
1      63       55.541
2      64       55.620     -1    -0.078173    0.0887 0.7669
```

Unsurprisingly, the covariate x_3 can be discarded, with the same high p-value as before, and the reduced model explains the data as good as the full model. The next candidates for reduction are x_2 and x_2^2, so we delete these two covariates using m3 <- update(m2, ~ . − x2 − I(x2^2)), which yields

```
Call:
lm(formula = y ~ x1 + I(x1^2) + I(x3^2), data = d)

Residuals:
Min          1Q          Median       3Q          Max
-1.97562     -0.59584     -0.09701     0.70987     1.67002

Coefficients:
              Estimate    Std. Error   t value    Pr(> |t|)
(Intercept)   1.464151    0.565332     2.590      0.0118       *
x1            0.943416    0.207696     4.542      2.43e − 05 ***
I(x1^2)       0.006575    0.018555     0.354      0.7242
I(x3^2)       0.985192    0.016233     60.689     < 2e − 16 ***
---
Signif. codes:0 '***' 0.001 '**' 0.01 '*' 0.05 '.' 0.1 ' ' 1

Residual standard error: 0.9218 on 66 degrees of freedom
Multiple R-squared: 0.9843,          Adjusted R-squared: 0.9835
F-statistic: 1376 on 3 and 66 DF, p-value: < 2.2e-16
```

Continuing in the same fashion until all remaining covariates become significant, we find the minimal adequate model, which in this case claims that the resulting response can be explained by x_1 and x_3^2 plus the intercept. The covariate x_2 was found to have no influence on the response. The minimal adequate model is therefore

$$Y = \beta_0 + \beta_1 X_1 + \beta_6 X_3^2 + \varepsilon,$$

with estimated parameters $\hat{\beta}_0 = 1.3$, $\hat{\beta}_1 = 1.02$, and $\hat{\beta}_6 = 0.99$, which are very close to their true values $\beta_0 = \beta_1 = \beta_6 = 1$. To check the assumptions of homoscedacity and normal errors, we again give the residuals and the normal Q–Q-plot in Fig. 4.6; both look fairly good, there is no sign of any structure in the residuals and the normal quantiles fit the residuals' quantiles nicely, even in the tails.

Practical procedure for finding minimal models. The procedure taken in the above example already uses the main ideas for more general cases. Typically, we start with

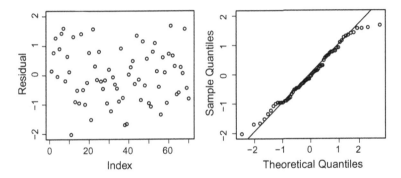

Fig. 4.6 Residuals (*left*) and normal Q–Q-plot (*right*) of fitted minimal adequate model, indicating homoscedacity and normal residuals, as assumed by the linear regression model

some plots like the demonstrated pairwise scatter plots to see which covariates have an influence, discover structure in the data, and find "curvature" in the relationships. We continue with a first full model containing all relevant covariates that showed other than fully random influence on the response. We also additionally include all covariates showing curvature by taking their square, square-root, logarithm, or similar. Looking at the summary, we iteratively delete the covariate with highest *p*-value until all parameters become significant. Using the anova() function, we check whether the reduced model is significantly worse than the non-reduced model. The last steps are repeated until we find the minimal adequate model.

It is important to note that this procedure, while quite successful in practice, does not necessarily finds the best minimal adequate model, as the *p*-values of all covariates are changed when one of it is discarded, and the final model often depends on the order in which variables are discarded. This becomes more pronounced if the covariates are dependent among each other, in which case the initial model should contain appropriate interaction terms.

4.4.4 Outliers

Least-squares based linear regression methods are not very robust towards *outliers*, which are points that are far from where they are expected to be. To measure the extend to which a particular data point influences the overall regression, we can remove each point successively, then fit the regression model without this point, and compute the overall standard deviation of this model. Points that change the overall standard deviation to a large extend then deserve special attention. Another measure to quantify the influence of a particular point on the overall regression is the *Cook's distance*, computed for the *j*th point by

Fig. 4.7 Linear regression in presence of an outlier (point marked x). The outlier has a very high leverage and the regression line is "pulled" towards it. The dashed line denotes the regression when ignoring the outlier

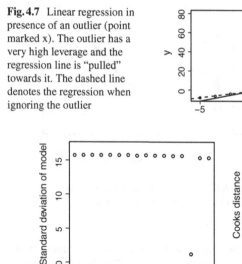

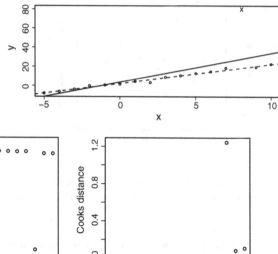

Fig. 4.8 Overall standard deviation (*left*) and Cook's distance (*right*) when fitting the linear regression without the corresponding sample point. The 14th sample point clearly stands out, requiring further attention when fitting the model

$$D_j = \frac{1}{m} \frac{\sum_{i=1}^{n} \left(\hat{y}_i - \hat{y}_{i \backslash j} \right)^2}{\hat{\sigma}^2},$$

where again n is the number of sample points, m is the number of covariates, and $\hat{\sigma}^2$ is the mean-squared error of the model. The two sets of predicted values are $\hat{y}_i$ for the model with all sample points and $\hat{y}_{i \backslash j}$ for the model without the jth sample point. This distance is given in one of the plots when using the `plot()` function on a fitted linear model and can also be computed using the function `cooks.distance()`.

Points that have a considerable influence on the parameter estimation are often called *influence points* or *leverage points*. They usually require special attention and one should always check how much the parameter values of the model change when ignoring such point.

Example 36 Consider the situation in Fig. 4.7, where a linear regression line is fitted to 16 data points, one of which is a clear outlier. The fitted line (solid) is "pulled" towards this outlier and both the intercept and the slope are considerably disturbed. In this case, the outlier is easily detected even by eye. Removing it from the data yields the dashed regression line, which shows an excellent fit. This is also reflected in the standard deviation, which is around 15.7 for all points but the outlier, and drops to 1.22 if the outlier is removed before estimating the parameters. The Cook's distances give a similar picture. Both measures are given for the 16 data points in Fig. 4.8.

While quite intuitive, the term *outlier* already implies that the proposed under-lying model is correct in the sense that all its assumptions, such as the linearity and homoscedacity, hold. If these assumptions are indeed correct, then leverage points can often be interpreted as incorrect measurement values. When values are recorded manually, a simple typo or a misplaced decimal point may already explain an unusual leverage point. In other cases, the measurement device might be incorrectly calibrated or failed to record a particular value, setting it to zero instead.

On the other hand, the underlying model may already be incorrect. For example, we may be using a linear regression model on data generated by a nonlinear rela-tion between covariate and response. Then, leverage points with, e.g., large Cook's distances, might simply be caused by wrong model assumptions and are not outliers in the sense of an incorrect measurement.

Example 37 Let us consider the following situation: we are given response data to a covariate x. The true response is a cubic function of the covariate, and the correct model is

$$Y = \beta_0 + \beta_1 X^3.$$

We now instead try to estimate the parameters of the regression model

$$Y = \beta_0 + \beta_1 X$$

using the data. This model neglects all the curvature, and we fit a straight line to the data. The resulting parameter estimates seem to look good; the slope parameter is significant and a good overall p-value for the model is achieved.

```
Call:
lm(formula = y ~ x)

Residuals:
Min             1Q          Median     3Q         Max
-590.255        -238.004    1.025      295.897    721.400

Coefficients:
                Estimate    Std. Error t value    Pr(> |t|)
(Intercept)     48.63       104.91      0.464      0.65
x               126.83      20.00       6.340      1.83e - 05  ***
---
Signif. codes: 0 '***' 0.001 '**' 0.01 '*' 0.05 '.' 0.1 ' ' 1

Residual standard error: 368.9 on 14 degrees of freedom
Multiple R-squared: 0.7417,          Adjusted R-squared: 0.7232
F-statistic: 40.19 on 1 and 14 DF, p-value: 1.829e-05
```

The overall fit is given by the solid line in Fig. 4.9 (left), with an analysis of its leverage points in Fig. 4.9 (right). However, the points with high leverage are

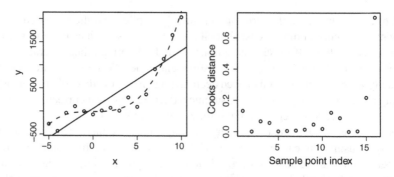

Fig. 4.9 *Left* Fit of linear model $Y = \beta_0 + \beta_1 X$ to function $y = 2 + 2x^3 + \varepsilon$ (*solid line*). The *dashed line* shows the fit of a cubic polynomial. *Right* Cook's distances as influence measures of straight-line model on the data

clearly not "outliers" in the sense of incorrect measurements, but are artifacts from our attempt to fit a straight line to a curved dataset. A more detailed inspection of the residuals and the fit is indicated and higher powers of the covariate such as x^2 and x^3 need to be added to the model. Fitting the correct model y ~ I(x^3) yields the dashed line in Fig. 4.9 (left), which shows an excellent fit.

4.4.5 Robust Regression

Least-squares estimation of regression parameters can be very sensitive to the presence of even a small number of outliers in the data. Therefore, the question for more robust methods naturally arises and we will very briefly present two alternatives to least-squares estimation that are less sensitive to outliers and have high breakdown points: the RLM approach tries to robustly fit a linear model using so-called M-estimators, while the LQS approach relies on resistant regression by picking only "good" points for the estimation. We can not present the details of these two approaches in this book, but both are conveniently implemented in the MASS package of R and can be called by rlm() and lqs(); these implementations can again be used using formulas, just like the lm() function for least-squares regression: rlm(y ~ x) and lqs(y ~ x) will do all the heavy lifting for us. They both encompass several different methods each, and work mainly by using order statistics for estimation and weighting schemes to detect and down-weight points with high leverage. For the two above examples of a true linear function and a cubic function, the fitted regression lines are shown in Fig. 4.10. For the linear data, the outlier clearly does not influence the regression line anymore and a very good fit is achieved with both methods, basically by ignoring the outlier or giving it a very low weight in the estimation. The estimated models are almost identical for both estimations. Using an incorrect model like the straight line for the cubic data, both methods will fail to

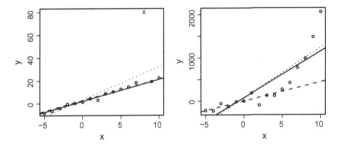

Fig. 4.10 Robust linear regression models of the linear (*left*) and cubic (*right*) dataset using the R function `rlm()` (solid) and `lqs()` (*dashed*). For the linear case, the two regressions are almost identical, but they differ substantially in the cubic case. The *dotted lines* indicate the non-robust fit using `lm()`

give a good explanation of the data, as shown in Fig. 4.10 (right). The two estimated models are very different, however, due to the different way the methods ignore and down-weight what seem to be outliers. For comparison, the non-robust least-squares estimates are also given in both cases.

4.5 Analysis-of-Variance

Using ideas very similar to linear regression of a metric response on metric covariates, we can also analyze the influence of categorial covariates on a metric response by ANOVA. There is a very rich theory on ANOVA, but we will only be concerned with the basic ideas and methods. In particular, we only discuss the case of one covariate.

4.5.1 Problem Statement

We consider one categorial covariate X and a metric response Y. In the context of ANOVA, the covariate X is called a *factor* and its different possible categories are called *factor levels*. We are interested in the question whether the different factor levels have an influence on the response or not, and whether these influences are substantially different for the different factor levels. Each factor level is claimed to give a particular response. Again, the response is subject to noise, so the same factor level may lead to different response values, spread around a certain value. Let us look into an example to make these considerations more concrete.

Example 38 We want to test the effect of different growth media (that is, mixtures of different nutrients) on the growth of cells. There are three different media: *A, B,* and a control medium, and *A, B* are both tested in a low and a high concentration. Thus,

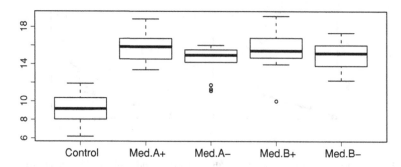

Fig. 4.11 Boxplot of cell growth response values for the control and two different media (A/B) with two concentrations (high/low) each

the covariate X is a factor with 5 levels, one for each possible medium. For each factor level (each medium), several experiments are conducted and the cell growth is recorded, which yields a metric response to the categorial covariate. A convenient way to visualize the influence of the factor levels on the response is the boxplot, which can easily be generated using `boxplot(growth ~ medium, data = d)` and is shown in Fig. 4.11. The first impression of this plot is that both A and B seem to have a considerable effect on the growth, but that there is no difference between them. The concentration of each medium also seems to have little to no effect. The main part of our discussion of ANOVA will revolve around making these impressions quantitative.

Formally, let us consider a factor X with k factor levels and assume that we have n_i observations for the ith level. Then, the ANOVA model is

$$Y_{ij} = \mu_i + \varepsilon_{ij}, \quad i = 1 \ldots k, \quad j = 1 \ldots n_i,$$

where Y_{ij} is the jth measured response for factor level i, μ_i is the true mean value for this level and ε_{ij} is the associated measurement error, which is again assumed to have mean zero and constant but unknown variance for all levels. Often, we again assume the error to have a normal distribution as well.

We can derive an equivalent model by replacing the factor level means μ_i by an overall mean μ_0 and the difference $\alpha_i = \mu_i - \mu_0$ of each level mean to the overall mean, yielding

$$Y_{ij} = \mu_0 + \alpha_i + \varepsilon_{ij}.$$

In essence, the ANOVA model claims that the undisturbed response at factor level i would take the value μ_i. Due to the error perturbing the measurement, measured values Y_{ij} spread around the value μ_i. The ANOVA is then performed to answer the question whether or not the factor level has an influence on the outcome and if so, which factor levels yield different outcomes. This in mainly a question whether the mean values of k levels differ significantly or not and in this sense, ANOVA can be seen as an extension of t-test procedures to more than two groups.

4.5.2 Parameter Estimation

In close resemblance to the linear regression, our first task is to estimate the various parameters of the ANOVA model. Let $n = \sum_i n_i$ be the total number of sample points from all levels. The estimators for the overall and the individual factor level means are then the arithmetic means taken over the corresponding sample points. The differences in means are estimated as the difference of the estimators, and we can also estimate the variance in the data in the straightforward way.

We therefore derive the estimators

$$\hat{\mu}_0 = \bar{y} = \frac{1}{n} \sum_{i=1}^{k} \sum_{j=1}^{n_i} y_{ij},$$

$$\hat{\mu}_i = \bar{y}_i = \frac{1}{n_i} \sum_{j=1}^{n_i} y_{ij},$$

$$\hat{\alpha}_i = \hat{\mu}_0 - \hat{\mu}_i,$$

$$\hat{\sigma}^2 = \frac{1}{n-k} \sum_{i=1}^{k} \sum_{j=1}^{n_i} \left(y_{ij} - \bar{y}_i \right)^2.$$

Because we estimate the variance from k different factor levels, the correct degrees of freedom are $n - k$.

4.5.3 Hypothesis Testing

For testing the various hypotheses on the influence of the factors, we can apply the same general ideas as for the linear regression analysis. In particular, we can decompose the total variation SS_{tot} in the data, given by

$$SS_{tot} = \sum_{i=1}^{k} \sum_{j=1}^{n_i} \left(y_{ij} - \bar{y} \right)^2$$

into the variation explained by the ANOVA model, and the remaining unexplained variation. In ANOVA, the explained variation is the *between-groups-variation*, caused by the different means for each factor level. It is calculated as the sum of squared differences of group (i.e., factor level) means to the overall mean, scaled by the appropriate number of samples in each group.

$$SS_{between} = \sum_{i=1}^{k} n_i \left(\bar{y}_i - \bar{y} \right)^2.$$

The remaining unexplained variation is the *within-group-variation* that measures how much the data from the same group disperses around the corresponding group mean.

$$SS_{within} = \sum_{i=1}^{k} \sum_{j=1}^{n_i} \left(y_{ij} - \bar{y}_i\right)^2.$$

The total variation is then again composed of the sum of between- and within-group-variation:

$$SS_{tot} = SS_{between} + SS_{within}.$$

As for the linear regression, the total variation is constant and independent of an ANOVA model, but the contributions of the within- and the between-group-variations to the total variation depend on the estimated parameters of the ANOVA model, allowing us to compare different models.

The global hypothesis. Again, the boldest hypothesis we might want to test is the global null hypothesis that none of the factor levels has an influence on the response. If this hypothesis is not rejected, the model does not explain any of the variation in the data. The hypothesis is

$$H_0 : \mu_1 = \cdots = \mu_k,$$

which is also equivalent to $H_0 : \alpha_1 = \cdots = \alpha_k = 0$, i.e., no difference in the expected response to the factor levels. Although we want to test the equality of group means, the test statistic is in fact based on comparing the between-group-variation $SS_{between}$ to the within-group-variation SS_{within}. Dividing each by their corresponding degrees of freedom, this ratio has an F-distribution, provided that the errors ε_{ij} are normally distributed. The test statistic is thus

$$F = \frac{SS_{between}/(k-1)}{SS_{within}/(n-k)},$$

and with $F \sim F(k-1, n-k)$, we reject H_0 at level α, if $F > F_{1-\alpha}(k-1, n-k)$.

Here is how this works: if the variation of response values in one group is similar to the overall variation, this indicates that these values can not be separated from the other groups. If, however, the variation in the group is much smaller than the overall variation, this means these values are more compact and have a distinct location within the overall data, making it easy to spot response values of this group. The two situations are depicted in Fig. 4.12: if the response values are comparatively compact for each group, and the groups are different, the within-group-variations are small compared to the between-group-variations (left panel). Conversely, similar within- and between-group-variations lead to many similar response values of different groups, making it difficult to distinguish them (right panel).

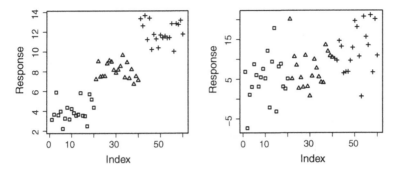

Fig. 4.12 *Left* Small within-group-variation ($SS_{within} = 54.93$) and large between-group-variation ($SS_{between} = 637.2$) indicate good separation of the groups. Shown are three factor levels with group means $\mu_1 = 4$ *(square)*, $\mu_2 = 8$ *(triangle)*, $\mu_1 = 12$ *(cross)*, and an error variance of $\sigma^2 = 1$, where group membership is indicated by different symbols. *Right* High within-group variation indicates bad separation and/or very high error variance ($SS_{within} = 1602.35$ and $SS_{between} = 556.24$). The same factor levels as before are used, but the error variance is now $\sigma^2 = 30$ and estimated as $\hat{\sigma}^2 = 28.11$

Example 39 Let us test the global hypothesis for the example of cell growth in five different media. The global null hypothesis states that the medium does not cause any difference and thus the average cell growth is the same for all five conditions. We get the data as a table with two columns, the first containing the measured growth value (a number), the second the factor level (here, a simple name). To get an impression of how this data looks like, a selected subset of the rows are given below:

```
     growth      medium
1    11.364981   Control
7     9.179241   Control
17   11.093238   Med.A-
41   15.848123   Med.A+
52   15.137522   Med.B-
59    9.982484   Med.B+
```

Once the data is established, we can formalize the model using the same R formulas as for the linear regression and simply apply the function `aov()` instead of `lm()`. Here, we compute the ANOVA of the response `growth` with respect to the factor `medium` on the data d:

```
model <- aov(growth ~ medium, data = d)
```

The `summary()` function is used to give the *ANOVA table*

```
            Df   Sum Sq   Mean Sq   F value   Pr(> F)
medium       4   456.70   114.17    34.920    1.495e − 15 ***
Residuals   65   212.52   3.27
---
Signif. codes: 0 '***' 0.001 '**' 0.01 '*' 0.05 '.' 0.1 ' ' 1
```

The column Df contains the degrees of freedom of the factor and the residuals, the columns Sum Sq and Mean Sq contain the sum of squares and the mean sum of squares (variation). The value Mean Sq of the Residuals is the pooled variance of the data, and the first row gives us the result of the global null hypothesis test. As indicated by the very low p-value, at least one of levels of the factor medium does significantly influence the response growth.

Contrasts While the global hypothesis is a first check to decide whether the factor has any influence at all, we are often interested in a more detailed analysis to see which factor levels have influence and whether the influences of the different levels are significantly different. For this, we need to be able to test subsets of factor levels against each other and formally state hypotheses like "the first and second level of the factor differ from each other" and "the first and second level might not differ, but both differ from the third". An elegant and powerful way to do this is by means of *linear contrasts*. A linear contrast is a weighted sum of the expected response to the factor levels

$$\Psi_C = \sum_{i=1}^{k} c_i \mu_i,$$

where $C = (c_1, \ldots, c_k)$ are any numbers that sum to zero: $c_1 + \cdots + c_k = 0$. Let us assume that we want to test the hypothesis that the factor levels i and j yield the same response, which we can write as $H_0 : \mu_i - \mu_j = 0$. This hypothesis can be recast in terms of a linear contrast by setting the contrast values $c_i = +1, c_j = -1$ and $c_l = 0$ for all other levels. The contrast then reads

$$\Psi_C = \mu_i - \mu_j,$$

and we test the equivalent hypothesis $H_0 : \Psi_C = 0$. The problem is thus transformed from testing combinations of factor levels against each other to testing whether a function of the group means (the contrast) is zero. For performing this test, we need to find an estimate for the contrast Ψ_C and to establish its distribution under the null hypothesis.

Estimating the contrast is again straightforward: with the c_i given, we can simply plug in the estimators for the group means to get the estimator for the contrast as

$$\hat{\Psi}_C = \sum_{i=1}^{k} c_i \bar{y}_i.$$

We already saw that if we use an estimator as a test statistic, we can use the $(1-\alpha)$-confidence interval of the estimator to get the corresponding rejection region of the test at level α: testing whether the contrast is zero at the test level α is equivalent to checking if the value zero is contained in the corresponding $(1 - \alpha)$-confidence interval of the estimate. This CI is given by the usual form

$$\text{CI}_\alpha = \hat{\Psi}_C \pm S_\alpha \widehat{\text{se}}(\hat{\Psi}_C),$$

where the standard error of the estimator is given by

$$\widehat{\text{se}}(\hat{\Psi}_C) = \hat{\sigma} \sqrt{\sum_{i=1}^{k} \frac{c_i^2}{n_i}},$$

as $\text{Var}(\hat{\Psi}_C) = \sum_i c_i^2 \text{Var}(\bar{y}_i)$ and $\text{Var}(\bar{y}_i) = \hat{\sigma}^2/n_i$. Testing the difference of two levels i, j is equivalent to a t-test, which would give us the quantile $S_\alpha = t_\alpha(v)$ with corresponding degrees of freedom v. However, using contrasts often means that we simultaneously perform several such pair-wise tests and thus need to correct for multiple testing. While the Bonferroni-correction works for a small number of contrast, another option is to use *Scheffé's-quantile*

$$S_\alpha = \sqrt{(k-1)F_{1-\alpha}(k-1, n-k)}.$$

The test at level α for a contrast Ψ_C is then:

$$\text{Reject} \quad H_0 : \Psi_C = 0 \quad \text{if} \quad 0 \notin \text{CI}_\alpha.$$

Setting up a contrast in the general case is very easy with the following rules:

- Setting the contrast value c_i to zero excludes the corresponding factor level.
- Factor levels with same sign for c_i are lumped into one group.
- Factor levels with different signs are contrasted, i.e., their means are compared.
- Overall, the contrast values c_i must sum to zero.

Let us look at a longer example, where we analyze the impact of the various media on the cell growth and try to figure out whether medium A and medium B differ from each other and from the control, and whether high versus low concentrations have an effect.

Example 40 From the last example, we know that the ANOVA model can explain the data with good p-value. In order to see the contribution of each factor level to this explanation, we can use the `summary.lm()` function.

```
Call:
aov(formula = growth ~ medium, data = d)

Residuals:
Min              1Q           Median        3Q           Max
-5.5530          -1.2744      0.2174        1.2053       3.6179

Coefficients:
                Estimate     Std. Error  t value    Pr(> |t|)
(Intercept)     9.1693       0.4669       19.640     < 2e - 16     ***
mediumMed.A+    6.7843       0.6405       10.591     8.62e - 16 ***
mediumMed.A-    5.1105       0.6852       7.459      2.67e - 10 ***
mediumMed.B+    6.3662       0.6719       9.474      7.30e - 14 ***
mediumMed.B-    5.6872       0.7178       7.923      3.99e - 11 ***
---
Signif. codes: 0 '***' 0.001 '**' 0.01 '*' 0.05 '.' 0.1 ' ' 1

Residual standard error: 1.808 on 65 degrees of freedom
Multiple R-squared: 0.6824,          Adjusted R-squared: 0.6629
F-statistic: 34.92 on 4 and 65 DF, p-value: 1.495e-15
```

The reported p-values of the four factor levels correspond to the difference of the factor level to the first factor level, i.e., the control. As expected from the first visual inspection of the data, all four differences of high A to the control, low A to the control and so forth are highly significant, indicating that using any medium yields better growth than using the control medium. However, the values do not allow us to see whether the concentrations have different effects, for example. We therefore want to test the following hypotheses:

1. control vs. other media. The claim is that the effect of the other media differs from the control. We formulate this by giving a contrast of +4 to the control, and -1 to each of the four other levels, thus $C = (4, -1, -1, -1, -1)$.
2. Medium A and medium B differ. We can ignore the control here, and group the two concentrations by choosing $C = (0, 1, 1, -1, -1)$.
3. High and low concentrations of A have different effect: $C = (0, -1, 1, 0, 0)$.
4. High and low concentrations of B have different effect: $C = (0, 0, 0, -1, 1)$.

These contrasts are simultaneously set up in R using the command

contrasts(d\$medium) <- cbind(c(4, -1, -1, -1, -1), c(0, 1, 1, + - 1, -1), c(0, -1, 1, 0, 0), c(0, 0, 0, -1, 1))

which yields the *contrast matrix*

```
> contrasts(d$medium)
            [, 1]    [, 2]    [, 3]    [, 4]
Control      4        0        0        0
Med.A+      -1        1       -1        0
Med.A-      -1        1        1        0
Med.B+      -1       -1        0       -1
Med.B-      -1       -1        0        1
```

This matrix is attached to the factor medium in the data frame d, and we can apply it by simply creating a new model with aov

```
model2 <- aov(growth ~ medium, data = d)
```

which yields the summary

```
Call:
aov(formula = growth ~ medium, data = d)
```

Residuals:

Min	1Q	Median	3Q	Max
−5.5530	−1.2744	0.2174	1.2053	3.6179

Coefficients:

	Estimate	Std. Error	t value	Pr(> |t|)	
(Intercept)	13.95894	0.21841	63.912	$< 2e - 16$	***
medium1	−1.19741	0.10562	−11.337	$< 2e - 16$	***
medium2	−0.03967	0.24681	−0.161	0.8728	
medium3	−0.83691	0.33310	−2.512	0.0145	*
medium4	−0.33948	0.36427	−0.932	0.3548	

```
Signif. codes: 0 '***' 0.001 '**' 0.01 '*' 0.05 '.' 0.1 ' ' 1
```

```
Residual standard error: 1.808 on 65 degrees of freedom
Multiple R-squared: 0.6824,          Adjusted R-squared: 0.6629
F-statistic: 34.92 on 4 and 65 DF, p-value: 1.495e-15
```

The first row gives again the global hypothesis that the factor levels give different response values. The second to fifth row give the results of the four contrasts attached to the data frame; only the difference of the control to the two other media is significant, whereas none of the comparisons between the non-control media shows a significant difference for $\alpha = 0.01$. To simplify the model, we can therefore continue our analysis by lumping the four non-control factor levels into a single new factor level by

```
medlumped <- d$medium
levels(medlumped)[2 : 5] <- "medium"
d$medium < medlumped
```

We again estimate the parameters for this new ANOVA model with only two factor levels and compare it to the original full model using the anova() function. The two models do not have significantly different explanatory power (at level $\alpha = 0.1$) and we found the minimal model explaining the data.

```
Analysis of Variance Table

Model 1: growth ~ medium
Model 2: growth ~ medium
     Res.Df    RSS       Df    Sum of Sq    F        Pr(> F)
1    65        212.52
2    68        236.00    -3    -23.480      2.3938   0.07639.
---
Signif. codes: 0 '***' 0.001 '**' 0.01 '*'0.05 '.' 0.1 ' ' 1
```

The most simple explanation of the observed responses to the various factor levels is thus only the difference between the control and *any* medium and we found that there is no difference between the two media, nor between a medium in low or high concentration.

4.6 Interpreting Error Bars

We conclude our investigation with a brief discussion of a common technique to find differences in the influences of factor levels on a response from plots of the data. In practice, the effect of a factor on a response is often not reported by giving the results of an ANOVA, but rather by plotting bar-graphs of the response, with one bar per factor level. The height of each bar then corresponds to the estimated mean value of the group and an error bar is provided. Sometimes, it is then argued that whenever two error bars overlap, the difference of the two groups is not significant, whereas if the bars do not overlap, the difference is significant. This, however, is only true for very particular choices of error bars under the strong additional assumption of normally distributed data in each group.

Standard deviations. The most common choice for error bars is to plot intervals of length corresponding to one standard deviation in each direction. Apart from the problem that very different data can give the same bar-plot (recall Sect. 1.8.4), knowing the mean and standard deviation does not allow inference of differences in the means. This is because the standard deviation represents the dispersion of values in the data, but not the uncertainty in the estimated means. This error bar is thus *descriptive*, but not *inferential*.

Confidence intervals. An option to derive inferential error bars is to compute the 95%-confidence intervals for each group mean and use their lengths as the lengths of the error bars. We know that the true value of a group mean is contained in the confidence interval of its estimate with probability $1 - \alpha$. If the confidence intervals of two estimated group means do not overlap, we can therefore safely infer that the two means are significantly different because the probability of them having the same value is lower than α. However, nothing can be said if two bars do overlap; thus, we can only infer different, but not equal group means using this method.

Standard errors. Alternatively, we can use the standard errors of the estimated group means. If we again denote by $\hat{\sigma}$ the standard deviation of the response, taken over all factor levels, we already know that the estimated standard error for the mean $\bar{y}_i$ of group i is $\widehat{se}(\bar{y}_i) = \hat{\sigma}/\sqrt{n_i}$ (the confidence interval then has length $2t_{1-\alpha/2}(n_i)\widehat{se}(\bar{y}_i)$). Let us recall that the difference $\mu_i - \mu_j$ of two group means is significant at the level α if

$$\left|\frac{\bar{y}_i - \bar{y}_j}{\widehat{se}(\bar{y}_i - \bar{y}_j)}\right| > t_{1-\alpha/2}(n_i + n_j - 2).$$

If the sample sizes n_i and n_j for the two groups are large enough, we know that $t_{0.975}(n_i + n_j - 2) \approx 2$ is a good approximation of the t-quantiles for $\alpha = 0.05$. Thus, the means are significantly different if they are more than twice the standard error of the estimated difference apart. The problem is that the standard error of the difference depends on the two groups that we compare and we can only give error bars that are valid for a particular pair of groups. However, this standard error is always smaller than the sum of the two standard errors of the individual means, because the variance of the difference is the sum of the variances:

$$\widehat{se}(\bar{y}_i - \bar{y}_j) = \sqrt{\frac{\hat{\sigma}^2}{n_i} + \frac{\hat{\sigma}^2}{n_j}}$$

$$\leq \sqrt{\frac{\hat{\sigma}^2}{n_i} + \frac{\hat{\sigma}^2}{n_j} + 2\frac{\hat{\sigma}}{\sqrt{n_i}}\frac{\hat{\sigma}}{\sqrt{n_i}}} = \sqrt{\left(\frac{\hat{\sigma}}{\sqrt{n_i}} + \frac{\hat{\sigma}}{\sqrt{n_j}}\right)^2}$$

$$= \widehat{se}(\bar{y}_i) + \widehat{se}(\bar{y}_j).$$

Therefore, we can use the individual standard errors for the means (one per group), but by doing so overestimate the standard error of the difference. This still allows us to infer that there is no significant difference (at the 5%-level) of any two group means if their corresponding error bars overlap. However, non-overlapping bars do not allow to infer a significant difference.

Least-significant difference (LSD). In the special case that each group has the same sample size, so $n_1 = \cdots = n_k$, the standard error of the differences

$$\widehat{se}(\bar{y}_i - \bar{y}_j) = \sqrt{\frac{\hat{\sigma}^2}{n_i} + \frac{\hat{\sigma}^2}{n_j}} = \sqrt{2\frac{\hat{\sigma}^2}{n_i}} = \sqrt{2}\frac{\hat{\sigma}}{\sqrt{n_i}},$$

is the same for all pairs i,j of groups. From this, we derive the LSD as LSD $= t_{1-\alpha/2}\sqrt{2}\frac{\hat{\sigma}}{\sqrt{n_i}}$. Using a length of LSD/2 for each arm of the error bar, this allows us to infer that there is no significant difference between the means of any two groups if the corresponding bars overlap and also that there is a significant difference between them if their corresponding bars do not overlap.

4.7 Summary

Regression analysis allows us to study the influence of one or several covariates on a response. If all variables are metric, we can perform a linear regression and estimate parameters either by a least-squares or by a robust RLM or LQS approach.

Confidence intervals for predicted values also depend on the distance of the new covariate value to those used for estimation.

Decomposing the total variation of the model into explained and unexplained variation allows us to use F-tests to discard covariates.

ANOVA lets us simultaneously compare several means by regressing a response on a factor with several levels. We test combinations of levels using F-tests on linear contrasts.

For normally distributed samples, we can visually infer differences in factor levels from overlaps in appropriate error bars.

Reference

1. Crawley, M.J.: Statistics – An Introduction using R. Wiley (2005)

Index

H.-M. Kaltenbach, *A Concise Guide to Statistics*, SpringerBriefs in Statistics,
DOI: 10.1007/978-3-642-23502-3, © Hans-Michael Kaltenbach 2012